What others are saying about

Sign Language of the Soul

"There is a biblical quotation, 'We're strange and wondrously made.' Dr. Schusterman makes newly rediscovered ancient concepts available to share. Read it with understanding that grows as you do."

GEORGE GOODHEART, DC, DIBAK
FOUNDER AND DEVELOPER OF APPLIED KINESIOLOGY

"Dale Schusterman has written a fascinating and helpful method for learning how you can help yourself as a soul, a whole person. The understanding he gives to the mystical traditions of healing are valuable insights which combine modern science and these methods. Reading and using these insights will allow the scientific minded as well as those on a Spiritual quest to gain greater understanding, health and wholeness. Sign Language of the Soul can help kinesiologists, biomedical practitioners and bodywork therapists be more effective personally and with their clients and patients."

JOHN F. THIE, DC AUTHOR OF *TOUCH FOR HEALTH*, FOUNDING CHAIRMAN
INTERNATIONAL COLLEGE OF APPLIED KINESIOLOGY, DIRECTOR PRAYER
AND HEALING MINISTRIES MALIBU UNITED METHODIST CHURCH

"I have long been impressed with Dr. Schusterman's creativity and his ability to penetrate both physiological and spiritual complexities. Now, he has culled truths from each and integrated them into a simplified, workable system that can help us to better understand our patients and ourselves."

WALTER H. SCHMITT, DC, DIBAK, DABCN

"Dr. Dale Schusterman has investigated and elucidated many of the most subtle and effective systems and modalities for promoting healing and well-being. He offers a particularly important contribution by making the esoteric accessible and guiding us to apply this timeless wisdom in helping ourselves and others."

LARRY DOSSEY, MD, AUTHOR OF *HEALING BEYOND WORDS*,
REINVENTING MEDICINE, AND *HEALING WORDS*

"Sign Language of the Soul is especially recommended for providing readers with a six step plan for activating the "Tree of Life" process of personal healing and balance. A welcome addition to Alternative Medicine, Judaic Studies, Metaphysical Studies, and Kabbalah Studies reference collections and reading lists, Sign Language of the Soul is commended as being a truly seminal and expertly presented work."

MIDWEST BOOK REVIEWS

"Dale Schusterman's ingenious healing techniques have been a vital part of my personal wellness program for decades. In Sign Language of the Soul, he's able to share his brilliance in a remarkably simple, effective, do-it-yourself therapy plan that can restore your physical well-being while heightening your body-soul connection. This is holistic 'first-aid' at its finest!"

TERAH KATHRYN COLLINS
AUTHOR OF THE WESTERN GUIDE TO FENG SHUI

"At last, a sure method to experience inner balance before interacting with others. This book covers amazing correlations between the creation patterns that civilizations have pondered for generations. A book to stretch your thinking—use simply or delve into your deepest inner being."

MARILYN ADAMS, L. AC.

"I found Sign Language of the Soul to be a fascinating look at the interplay between some of the more esoteric healing modalities in the context of current alternative care. This book is an excellent representation of the concepts that have come out of Dr. Schusterman's research and the methods that can be used to apply them."

TOM ROGOWSKEY, DC, DIBAK

"I believe Dr. Schusterman's healing techniques constitute the blueprint for the maintenance of the health and balance of the body by natural medicine. Dr. Schusterman's healing methods bring immediate and amazing results, giving one an optimal quality of health and youthfulness."

SANDRA E. COPE, DESIGNER AND MANUFACTURER
OF ALOE SPECTRUM NATURAL SKIN CARE

"With profound, yet simple insights, Dr. Schusterman offers an understanding of the macrocosm and microcosm within each one of us. Anyone who wishes to look beyond the superficial constructs of the material world and into the underlying forces/energies of creation should read this marvelous book."

MARK SMITH, DC, DABCN

"This is truly extraordinary work—the deepest technique I have ever learned. It actually addresses the core/cellular levels of one's issues; be it physical, emotional, mental or spiritual. Dr. Schusterman's balancing system is groundbreaking and is the new wave of vibrational medicine!"

JANET QUATE, LPT

"I have known Dr. Schusterman for over 15 years as a care provider, and he has been spectacularly successful. I have always wondered what he is doing that is so helpful and effective. Well, now I know...his book offers insights, underlying philosophies, as well as practical techniques, all of which I as a patient can employ with myself and my wife. Thank you, Dr. Schusterman, for helping me help my wife get through chemotherapy more comfortably than with any of the currently available drugs!"

DON REISLER

"This is a very useful workbook with tremendously effective techniques. I am really enjoying using the *Sign Language of the Soul* with my clients, focusing first on their emotional or physical issue and then activating the tree of life... beautiful shifts happen."

JULIE LUTTER, L. AC.

Sign Language of the Soul
A Handbook for Healing
2nd Edition

Dr. Dale H. Schusterman

If you have any physical or psychological problems, consult a physician
before attempting the procedures in this book. These procedures are not
a substitute for proper medical care. The author and publisher assume
no responsibility for your health treatment program. Competent
health professionals should supervise the use of the methods taught
in this book.

Illustrations by Christine Felter
www.outsiderdesign.com

Library of Congress Cataloging-in-Publication Data

Schusterman, Dale H., 1951-
  Sign language of the soul: a handbook for healing, 2nd edition / by Dale
H.
Schusterman.
     p. cm.
Includes bibliographical references and index.
  ISBN 1-932133-05-4 (hardcover : alk. paper)
  1. Healing. 2. Touch--Therapeutic use. 3. Mind and body. 4. Mudråas
(Hinduism) I. Title.
  RZ999.S369 2003
  615.8'52--dc21
                              2003009134

Printed in the United States

Published by The Writers' Collective, Cranston, Rhode Island

Acknowledgments

This book has been incubating for almost two decades although the writing process has taken just over a year. Many people have touched my life in this time, so it would be impossible to mention them all. The material in this book is a product of love. Each time I became more aware of the love in my life, the work would expand. The key to accessing the deeper levels within the soul is to learn to open to the love that exists within us and to recognize that it is all around us as well. I am grateful to all the people who have touched my heart and have helped with this book. Some of them are listed here. The deepest love comes from my parents, Dan and Gloria Schusterman. My wife, Blanca, and daughter, Julia, are constant reminders of the love in my life. My dear friend Bobbi Garrett has been a source of great support and inspiration through the years. Marilyn Adams has been watching and supporting this work since the first mudra. I am very grateful to Christine Felter for designing the book and for her excellent illustrations that permeate it. Many thanks go to Suzi Tucker for her editing and guidance in the writing and publishing process. Thanks to Terah Kathryn Collins for her constant support and friendship. Leang Eap, Don Reisler, Tom Rogowskey, Mark Smith and Susan Ulfelder helped read the text for clarity and accuracy. I am ever grateful to George Goodheart and Walter Schmidt, Jr. for teaching me applied kinesiology and to Alan Beardall for teaching me the importance of hand positions in healing. Some of my many teachers, friends, and colleagues whom I wish to acknowledge are, Chris Astill-Smith, Rich Fischer, Cissy Garrett, Michael Gelb, Genevieve Haller, Stephan Hausner, Bert Hellinger, Marilyn Holbeck, Richard Miller, Janet Quate, Swami Shankarananda, Lawrence Steinhart, Linh Dieu Trang, John Ulfelder, and a special thanks to ABES_KIDS.

Contents

IV. Activating the Tree of Life

V. Balance

Final Thoughts

Appendixes

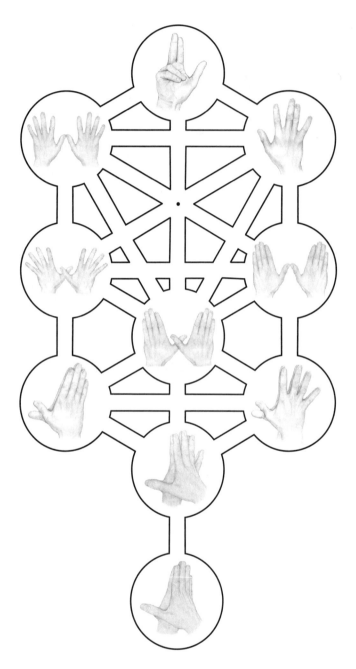

Sign Language of the Soul

"There are higher holier worlds than this one.
Obviously no one can know how many there are.
Nor can we be certain
That a certain rung of holy awareness
Is the same for different persons.
We only know that most of the time,
We are busy here,
Below the bottom one.
And that above the top one is the Nameless One,
The one named Ayn Sof, the One without end.
And that He comes down to us, as it were,
Like light poured down
Through some cascading waterfall.
And that we go up to Him
Through the same network,
Like salmon returning upstream to spawn.
But that whether like water down a fall
Or creatures swimming home,
By the time each reaches its destination
There is not much remaining.
Only a thin diluted version of what once started out.
So that what we see of Him here
Is dim.
And what He sees of us on high,
While very true to what we really are,
Might not look the way we do
To each other.
But in any case, ordinary souls like you and I are the link between
this world and the higher ones, shuttling back and forth, carrying
buckets of light in our heads."

Excerpt from Honey from the Rock: An Introduction to Jewish Mysticism – Special Anniversary
Edition © by Lawrence Kushner (Woodstock, VT: Jewish Lights Publishing). $15.95+$3.75 s/h.
Order by mail or call 800-962-4544 or on-line at www.jewishlights.com. Permission granted by
Jewish Lights Publishing, P.O. Box 237, Woodstock, VT 05091.

For Julia

Preface

My conscious inward journey began in 1971 after reading *Autobiography of a Yogi*, by Paramahansa Yogananda. I was a sophomore at the University of Michigan and experiencing many new ideas. This book, however, opened me up to an entirely new world of thinking. In my typical fashion, I jumped into yoga, meditation, and alternative diets with full zeal. Soon I was on the number 7 macrobiotic diet, eating only rice, and I was meditating for six or more hours a day. I thought I was on the crash course to enlightenment, but all I did was crash. The imbalance of my life soon caught up with me and I became ill. I was confused, emotionally off balance, and malnourished. In desperation, I put my name on a prayer list that was available at a meditation group I attended. That in itself was a big step for me. Within several hours, a person I had met only that morning took me to the home of a woman, a stranger to me, who was clairvoyant. The woman looked at me and told me that I had low back pain. When I asked her how she knew this, she told me that she could see "red in my aura." I asked her what an aura was. She explained it, and then said that she saw bones all around me and that I might become a chiropractor or osteopath. I was not sure what either of these terms really meant, but continued to listen. She steered me toward the Edgar Cayce readings as a way to involve me in a more balanced method of meditation and spiritual growth. The ascetic path I was on was too rigid for me, and although there are many balanced ways of following the Eastern path, I was not on one and a new approach was what I needed. I learned, from studying Cayce, that the important "spiritual work" includes balancing out negative attitudes and emotions, and healing one's relationships.

Reading Cayce also taught me about the possibilities of holistic healing. In the early 1970s, if you took vitamin C, people considered you a "health nut" and health-food stores were very hard to find. Nevertheless, I started studying all I could about nutrition and health. On my first visit to a chiropractor, I knew as soon as I walked into his office that this was what I would do with my life. I have never regretted the decision. During this time, I also followed every guru and psychic who came to town. Some were better than others, and a few were disasters. The function of a guru is to "dispel" the illusions of disciples. As it turns out, if they do not dispel your illusions, then they usually "dis-illusion" you. Either way, the illusions are dispelled. I learned the hard way the meaning of the statement from the mystical Qabalah, "God is the only guru, so get off your gatekeeper's back!"[1]

The development of an inner life has been paramount to me and my search has taken me through all the major religions and mystical traditions. I gradually learned, after some difficult lessons, how to be practical about these matters. One of the core teachings in all mystical systems is that for every step forward you take in spiritual understanding, you must take four or five steps forward in developing and balancing your personality toward humility, service to others, and similar goals. The true spiritual path lies in ordinary human experiences through relationships and family. We all have seen the harm inflicted by those who achieve power without the humility to handle it properly. Therefore, I resolved to learn as much as I could about different theories, systems, and concepts, but only use what I could verify and apply within my own understanding at any given time. The macrobiotic number 7 diet may be good for some people, but I wanted to know how to tell whether or not it was appropriate for me.

After my undergraduate studies, I attended chiropractic college. I was introduced to applied kinesiology, a new technique that would enable me to test the body directly to ascertain whether or not it needed something at any given time. The muscle-testing procedures provided me with a way to start working with the body in a cooperative fashion. I could test to see if a treatment would, or would not, enhance strength in the body. I could put a vitamin on the tongue and test to see if the body really needed it at that time. For instance, sometimes a supplement would test useful in the morning,

---

[1] Feldman, Daniel (2001). *Qabalah, The Mystical Heritage of the Children of Abraham*. Santa Cruz, CA: Work of the Chariot.

but not in the evening. It was possible to test a procedure to see if it was compatible with the body. These tools, in combination with my chiropractic knowledge, allowed me to help many people. It was also my key to finding balance in my own approach to health and inner clarity, as I could now distinguish between my mental concepts and the truth of the body.

Then, in October 1983, I had an inner experience that opened a completely new direction in my life. In essence, I was given a key to unlock the door to the spiritual current within me. My hands spontaneously moved into a special configuration that opened my body to the Tree of Life. Similar to the hand positions used in signing for the hearing impaired, this hand signal communicated something to and from my inner being (see Chapter 4). For years, I had studied every mystical path except the one at the core of my own Jewish religion. It was not until I began to plumb the roots of Judaism that I found the fulfillment I had been seeking. This book is the result of 20 years of studying Jewish mysticism known as the Kabbalah. This was not just a mystical exploration, although there were many such experiences along the way; it was a journey of self-discovery, self-healing, and awakening. I followed the energies that opened within me and each stage helped prepare me for the next one. I consulted a number of books, but mostly just to look at the charts and pictures. I did not delve into the written body of literature until recent years. Almost all of my early research was a product of inner experience as I explored the energies of the Tree of Life within my own system.

When I received the first hand sign in 1983, I thought that I had the key to the entire Kabbalah. In a sense, the key unlocked the door to the Tree of Life, but it has taken almost two decades to receive and understand the full set of hand signs presented in this book. Each new level would become accessible to me when I was ready for it, but not until I had integrated the previous level. In my deep inner contemplations, what allowed me to move to the next level of understanding was always the facing and overcoming of some internal block or resistance. It is necessary that all of us face the deep hurt, fear, guilt, doubt, and other complex issues of the human condition. Given this, Kabbalists should usually be at least 40 years of age and have a family before discussing these matters publicly. Of course, there are exceptions to this, however, the importance of the wisdom that comes from basic human life experience cannot be overstated, and it is not until we have reached middle age that we have had a chance to face many of our own deeper issues and have gained respect for the difficulty and complexity of life. It is my hope that those who study this material will be able to use it to help to bring light to their own areas of inner darkness.

These insights have also been helpful in my work with patients through the years. Much of my success as a chiropractic physician is a result of the healing energies of the Kabbalah that have opened within me. It is my desire to share these healing insights, principles, and methods with you. You do not need to be a physician to utilize the procedures taught in this book. Anyone can use them. However, you must not take on the role of physician with yourself or others if you are not qualified. Always maintain a broad perspective when dealing with self-balancing, or the treatment of others.

The procedures taught in this book are safe and can help almost anyone, but they are not medical treatments for serious conditions. Keep in mind that there is a time, and a place, for all types of healing. I still use chiropractic, nutritional approaches, detoxification methods, bioresonance, electro acupuncture, and family constellations when I work with patients. I also refer people to other physicians and therapists when necessary.

Those who strive to be healers should find these balancing procedures very useful. We must heed the adage "Healer, heal thyself" if we are to become healers for others. Therefore, if you are doing this work with others, you should regularly use the balancing procedures on yourself. Healing is more than a technique. It is the transference of love, energy, and compassion, along with knowledge and skill.

I continue to grow and develop new understandings of this amazing system (and myself) each day and do not claim to have any ultimate answers. I offer this material as the fruit of my own experience and ask that you take the information into your own personal laboratory to work with it and see how it helps your health, balance, and inner clarity.

The chapters that follow will detail how to do this. I wish you great success as you learn to "speak" a Sign Language of the Soul.

– Dale Schusterman

This second edition contains important revisions from the original book. New insights revealed that the addition of one mudra, along with activating the four doorways in the reverse order, would give a much deeper and simpler correction. As a result, there is no longer need for the balancing symbols, or the complex treatment protocols taught in the first edition.

Although advanced methods, which are taught in workshops, take this work to new heights, the methods described herein have broad application and produce wonderful results.

For those of you who are visual learners, a video is now available that demonstrates the methods described in this book. Go to www. SignLanguageoftheSoul.com for information on the video. While visiting the web site, check out the Vitruvian Man Healing exercise as well. Enjoy!

– Dale Schusterman
July 2007

INTRODUCTION

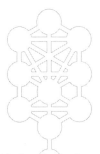

The main premise of this book is that the human body, and the energetic system that surrounds it, is a miniature replica of a larger, universal system. This is not a new concept, and it will be the subject of much discussion throughout the book. The procedures described here use knowledge of the anatomy of the universal system, or macrocosm, to understand how best to address the human system, or microcosm. You will learn specific ways to bring the human body-mind into alignment with the higher pattern, and this will enable you to develop a healing approach that can be applied to yourself or others. The tools you will use to tune the body-mind to its higher blueprint are hand signs or mudras, Hebrew and Sanskrit words, and the touching of special points on the body.

Through this work, you can balance many structural mis-alignments, energetic imbalances, and emotional traumas. In other words, you will find that spinal subluxations clear up, acupuncture meridians balance out, and emotional stresses literally cease to be a problem. However, these procedures are not a cure-all. They are highly effective in balancing a person, but they do not address all of a person's needs. People still require nutritional support, detoxification, structural support, life-style management, exercise and movement therapies, improved self-esteem, healthy relationships, and purpose in life. This includes the possible need for allopathic care.

Nevertheless, the procedures presented here can be of great value because they address the human system from a unique health perspective.

They rely on the wisdom of a fundamental blueprint that exists in the deeper levels of our being, the same blueprint as for the cosmos. Most people can benefit from several balancing sessions of the kind offered here, but the more consistently a person uses these procedures over time, the deeper the effect they have.

A special aspect of these procedures is that the individual receiving the balancing determines the direction the treatment takes. He or she is always in control of the process. The person directing the treatment simply follows, via manual muscle testing, the pathways that open up in the client. The interactive nature of this work allows the gradual, harmonious awakening and integration of these higher energies in the body.

These methods work equally well for people of all religious perspectives. The work is not about religion. It is about balancing the human body-mind in accordance with a cosmic blueprint. This approach is not the only way, or necessarily even the best way, to align the body to and with the subtle energy fields. It is one way.

In addition, although these procedures incorporate mystical teachings, their performance does not require mystical or psychic abilities. If you are a practitioner, your clients do not need to see or even know about the hand signs that you use in order for them to experience a positive outcome. Practically anyone who is open, focused, and able to follow the directions can activate the pathways. Although it is helpful to develop some skill in muscle-testing, this knowledge is not essential to do this work. Becoming proficient in muscle testing comes with experience and does not depend upon extraordinary ability. Healing is as much an art as it is a science.

Health

Health is more than the absence of symptoms; it is the presence of robust vitality in the physical body, emotional freedom, mental clarity, and an inner connection to something sacred. We are multidimensional beings, and all these areas need to be in harmony for us to be truly healthy. Millions of people each year now seek out complementary (holistic) therapies because they want all parts to be addressed in the healing process. These are nutritional or homeopathic therapies as well as body-centered therapies, such as chiropractic, massage, or craniosacral techniques. Other complementary therapies involve energy-balancing techniques, such as acupuncture, Reiki, Polarity Therapy, and Qi Gong. What you are about to study in this book is an approach to healing that grew out of my 25-year practice as a chiropractic physician, but is now a completely separate and distinct therapeutic system. This work acknowledges the inner being and it uses a spiritual blueprint to organize and implement the healing process.

This is not a new idea. Eastern cultures have systems of healing and balance based on esoteric cosmologies. Yoga, T'ai Chi, Qi Gong, and meridian therapy (acupuncture) all view human beings as part of a greater cosmic system. Yoga is based on the concepts of Tantric Hinduism. T'ai Chi, Qi Gong, and meridian therapy are based on the theory of the Tao, including the five elements and the yin and yang. These systems, all of which seek to bring people into harmony with higher forces, are effective for maintaining and enhancing health, and, in many cases, for curing disease.

The Western approach to health, on the other hand, looks at health from all of its physical perspectives. Western science has excelled in biochemistry, physiology, biomechanics, and many areas of psychology. Yet, as tremendous as this knowledge is, and as much as it has improved the quality of life and increased our longevity, it is incomplete without the spiritual component. This is why the complementary health movement in the West has embraced many of the Eastern systems.

What is little known is that there is a Western esoteric tradition that can provide us with specific healing methodologies. The paradigm presented here will associate many aspects of Jewish mysticism, known as Kabbalah, with the anatomy and physiology of the human body. Out of this integration come methods you can utilize to enhance health and inner balance. This Western wisdom tradition, although mystical

3

in nature, contains many references that relate this knowledge to the physical body. In fact, the human form is seen as a direct expression, or reflection, of the divine Being. Through this association, we can learn new ways to address and balance the human system. Since the map of the soul is the same for the body, one can literally navigate this map, the Tree of Life, within the body. This book will show you how.

Kabbalah

The term "Kabbalah" means tradition, or that which is received. Although the name Kabbalah dates back only to the 12th century, it is said that HaShem (literally, The Name), or God, originally taught it to Abraham when He formed His Covenant with him. This knowledge was passed on to each generation orally, from teacher to student, and was occasionally enhanced by the revelations of one of the prophets. Generally, the masses were 'protected' from its power, and although there have been various schools of Kabbalah over the centuries, most of them were secretive and reluctant to share their wisdom with the outside world.

Today, many people are awakening to this ancient wisdom, through books, teachers, and inner experience. The core texts of the Kabbalah are the *Torah*, *Sefer Yetzirah*, and the *Zohar*. Some people also include the *Talmud* and the *Bahir* in this list. In addition to these older texts, the last two decades have shown a proliferation of books on the Kabbalah, covering topics from health and spirituality, to particle physics.

Judaism traces its roots to the *Torah*, the first five books of the Jewish scripture. The Jewish bible also consists of the Prophets and the 11 books of the *Hagiographa*. Like all scriptural writing, the *Torah* can be interpreted on multiple levels. The Kabbalah provides an inner meaning or mystical interpretation of the Torah. The book of Genesis, the story of Exodus, and the vision of Ezekiel provide Kabbalists with some of their most important imagery.

4

One of the central Jewish mystical texts, the *Sefer Yetzirah*, or the *Book of Formation*, appeared sometime between the third and sixth centuries, but was not published until the mid-1500s. This short text contains the basis for much of Kabbalistic thought and it is integral to this book. It describes the stages and building blocks of creation. The correlation of the human body with these building blocks comes from this text, tying language to form and showing the essence of "as above, so below." Man/woman is a microcosm of a grand Creator and this relationship is evident in these teachings.

The *Zohar*, or *Book of Splendor*, is a multi-volume book that may stem from 13th century Spain, but is quite likely to have much earlier origins. It gives a mystical commentary on the Torah, and offers elaborate descriptions of the Tree of Life and the qualities of its various aspects.

Most modern books on the Kabbalah provide commentary and specific discussion on the early texts. The mysticism remains the same, but people of different levels of knowledge and degree of inner development provide their interpretation. Obviously, some of these observations are more useful than are others.

A book that has had a great influence on my own under-standing of the Kabbalah is *Qabalah, The Mystical Teachings of the Children of Abraham*, by Daniel Feldman of the Work of the Chariot (Qabalah indicates the mystical approach). The author makes this complex subject clear and intelligible. Any serious student of the Mysteries should read this book, which is universal in its presentation. You should consider it a companion book to this one, as it will enhance your understanding of the Kabbalistic material in this book. Much of the information from Feldman's book, including a downloadable PDF copy of his book, is also available online at www.workofthechariot.com. The specific letter pathways of the Tree of Life that Feldman describes are the ones used in this book. Of the many pathway correlations expounded by different authors, only Feldman's scenario tests to work in the body, as you will learn in Chapter 11.

I have chosen to write on the practical Kabbalah as my focus is on healing. I am not a rabbi, or a Hebrew scholar, and I claim no authority in these areas. My expertise is as a healer and chiropractic physician. Therefore, this book will emphasize how to use the design of the Kabbalistic Tree of Life to promote health and balance in the body-mind. This work serves to balance and integrate the human body-mind to the subtle multilayered structure of the soul. Moving through one's soul to the Mystery beyond is each person's personal journey. However, when the blocks are removed, it can help facilitate this process.

Mysticism

Imagine trying to describe the taste of a strawberry to someone who had never tasted fruit. No matter how rich your description, it will never quite match the experience. However, if a person hears your description and later on tastes the strawberry, the explanation will become meaningful. The same is true with mystical experience. Mysticism is the direct experience of spiritual reality. The only pathway to this knowledge is experience. Mystical teachings give rules and tools to help one safely access the inner realms, or they try to inspire with their stories and poetry. Once you have the experience, the words take on new meaning. There are cultural preferences and individual ways of expressing this inner knowledge, but, for the most part, they are all describing the same reality. No matter what language or metaphor one uses, a strawberry is still a strawberry. The major mystical teachings of the world include the Jewish Kabbalah, Hermetic Christianity, Gnosticism, Sufism (Islam), Tantric Hinduism, Taoism, and Buddhism. These teachings all describe the nature of our inner self and of God. They all say that our essential nature is holy and sacred, and that, at this level, we are one.

Although every term in the Kabbalah can be equated with a similar term in the other systems, the goal of this book is to show a clear, easy way to follow the divine pattern in the body based on the patterns found in the Kabbalah. References to Hindu Tantra and Eastern philosophy are important in certain phases of this work, but not from a religious perspective. This study of the interaction between the inner worlds and the human body should not be confused with the endorsement of any particular brand of religion.

What You Will Learn

The Kabbalah is a vast system of knowledge, covering all aspects of human experience; however, I focus primarily on how the patterns of the Tree of Life manifest in the body-mind and how to activate them. In the pages that follow, you will learn a unique, interactive approach to balancing the body-mind, based on this Western wisdom tradition. You will be able to apply these methods and immediately observe their effect, all under the guidance of the person's body with which you are working. This study will include coverage of the following:

1. A complete, yet concise, description of the different pathways of the Tree of Life
2. Where these pathways are located in the body and how to test them
3. A description of the four levels of existence and how they express in and through the body
4. Effective methods to balance the body-mind

There are many new concepts to learn, but you can master the actual application of these principles with minimal effort. These powerful tools, in the right hands, and guided by the right heart, can help people to greater health and inner awareness. They are also excellent self-help tools.

Format of the Book

Section I, "Physical Methods," sets the stage for understanding the healing process. There are certain limits and rules that are important to be aware of regarding these procedures. You will see how the Kabbalistic patterns manifest in the physical body, and you will learn a simple muscle test that will enable you to evaluate these patterns.

Section II, "Tools," begins to develop the methods used to tune

7

the body to the Tree of Life. You will start to learn a Sign Language of the Soul, including the hand signs (mudras) based on the Hebrew letter Shin, שׁ. These tools open the Kabbalistic patterns in the body. Chapter 7, "Resonance," will show how to use muscle testing to demonstrate that this is not just theory; it really works.

Section III, "Anatomy of the Tree of Life," describes just that. You will learn the various pathways of the Tree: the 10 Sefiroth, the 22 letter pathways, and the four worlds. We will work with multiple levels of the worlds and Chapter 9 will explain how to know which ones are active in the body.

In Section IV, "Activating the Tree of Life," you will learn a powerful centering procedure. Chapter 12 explores the different levels of the soul according to the Kabbalah. Here you will learn how to acknowledge the deeper aspects of the Tree. Chapters 13-16 develop the methods to activate the Tree of Life in the body. The summary of the Tree of Life activation can be found at the end of Chapter 16, pages 164-5.

Section V, "Balance," puts all the information to practical use. You will learn how to use the 10 Sefiroth mudras, or their corresponding body points to complete the healing process. You can also look at the illustration of the Tree of Life Mudras to accomplish the same thing (page iv).

Chapter 18 takes a deeper look at the healing process. You will learn how to bring hidden imbalances to the surface. Once revealed, they can be corrected with the Tree of Life activation, and one of the ten Sefiroth mudras.

"Final Thoughts" looks ahead to the next steps in the evolution of this work. The appendixes contain a synopsis of all the hand signs, words, and balancing procedures.

Finally, most chapters contain exercises to help you learn the principles of activating the different energy pathways in the body. It is best to do them with a partner. You are encouraged to spend some time on them, as it will greatly enhance your ability to understand and integrate this work.

There is a lot of material in this book and much of it will probably be new to you. Keep in mind, however, that the procedures are quite simple to perform. The Tree of Life activation process, summarized at the end of Chapter 16, takes less than a minute. You do not need to memorize everything in this book in order to learn the methods and obtain good results. Simply do the Tree of Life activation process and then look at Tree of Life mudra picture. Repeat the process until you no longer feel changes taking place.

A Chiropractor's Perspective

Even before entering chiropractic college, in 1973, I knew that there was more to understanding health and disease than traditional medicine, or even chiropractic, had to offer. I sensed that a sacred place existed within each individual and that it was always present, even in the most difficult situations. I also knew that discovering and acknowledging this special place in a person would create new opportunities to help. My job as a chiropractic physician was to correct imbalances in people's spines and extremities, yet I continued to seek out ways to enhance their well-being. I added numerous other therapies to my repertoire, including techniques found in applied kinesiology, such as cranial alignment, muscle balancing, meridian therapy, nutrition, the use of psychological affirmations, and so on. Yoga, Qi Gong, color, sound, and light therapies, and bioresonance, among others, also crossed my path.

Adding more therapies, however, did not satisfy my desire to touch a deeper place in my patients, although it did extend my treatment range. Then, in 1983, I received the first Kabbalistic hand sign (see Chapter 4). This began a new phase of my healing work. I applied this new knowledge to myself first, and then later to my patients. As the pathways of the Tree of Life unfolded within me, I not only resolved

9

many of my own issues, but found that I was able to do so for others as well. Chronic problems usually have deep roots that topical therapies, though palliative, are insufficient to correct. The new impulse that was developing within me, based on the Kabbalah, was what I had long been seeking.

I learned early in my chiropractic practice that telling people the correct way to eat, stand, sit, and think in order to enhance and preserve their health was successful only a small percentage of the time. Certainly, many people would listen to my advice and would benefit from it, but often those who really needed to listen and make positive changes in their lives were unable to translate it into positive action. A more effective approach to encouraging changes in lifestyle was not only to help them improve their immediate physical condition, but also to help them feel better about themselves. When we feel good, our self-image is healthy, our relationships are apt to be more fulfilling and fruitful, and we are likely to make good decisions. Many of us have it backwards. For example, many people believe that if they were to lose weight, they would be happy. Truthfully, if they find their inner happiness, the weight will more likely come off naturally. New life-style habits will be a by-product of their inner joy.

Chiropractors attempt to align the body to gravity. In other words, they align the structure so that it is mechanically sound while one is sitting, standing, and so on. I would never underestimate the benefit and importance of this. However, it has been my observation that we rely even more on being in alignment with our inner being than we do on gravity. Our body expresses the state of our soul even more than it reflects our relationship to gravity. When we are totally attuned with our inner selves, then we are firmly grounded in and on the earth. We feel great when we are mechanically aligned so that our posture is centered with gravity, but the results often do not last. Again, the inner pattern always surfaces eventually.

Both approaches to health are important. Everyone should avail themselves of a good spinal adjustment from time to time, and more

10

often if specific conditions require it. In addition, using procedures such as those found in this book will add tremendous depth and longevity to the spinal manipulations (or any other therapy) because they balance the deeper cause of the misalignments. When we balance the infrastructure, many other conditions disappear, and such balancing extends the benefit of any other therapies we might be using.

This book will teach you how to begin to balance the roots of the problems you experience with your health and in other areas of your life. You may experience complete alleviation of your condition. You may discover a new level of energy, inner clarity, and sense of well-being as you deal with life's challenges. The procedures will not fix everything, of course, but if you work with them for a while, the changes can be dramatic. It still amazes me to see obvious structural misalignments literally disappear as the result of a simple hand sign or by thinking or saying a word that causes the body to resonate to one of the frequencies of the Tree of Life. Likewise, a major life trauma can resolve just as easily. A simple attunement to the Tree of Life can create a profound effect that will last long after you close this book.

Betty

Betty, a 51-year-old social worker, came into my office seeking treatment for neck pain. She had a recent diagnosis of breast cancer and despite a successful lumpectomy, her oncologists wanted her to do radiation and chemotherapy, as a precaution against reoccurrence. Her family physician, along with several family members, were unsure if this was the best course of treatment for her. She was getting different advice from everyone. I suspected that her discomfort was actually related to her confusion and fear.

After a brief exam and discussion of her current health situation, I began her treatment. I used the hand signs to focus her to the frequencies of the Tree of Life and I observed the response in her body through the use of manual muscle testing. After six gentle corrections using the hand signs, her spine was pain free. Then I had her think about the choices she needed to make concerning her cancer treatment. Just thinking about it caused her muscle test to weaken. I applied the Sign Language of the Soul balancing procedures after each visualization of the stress. Six more gentle corrections enabled her to consider her choices, and the reactions of her family members, without weakening.

She left the office pain free and once again in control of her emotions and life. I did not interfere with her choice. It was more important to support her in making her own decisions. She never saw the hand signs I was using (it was not necessary) and was only aware of the gentle contact I made with her during the treatment. I was both grateful and pleasantly surprised by how easily her condition resolved.

The story on the previous page is one example of how the Sign Language of the Soul procedures work. Other vignettes are scattered throughout the book to help you understand the scope and power of the simple methods presented. Learning these procedures and how to creatively apply them will give you amazing tools for self-help and healing.

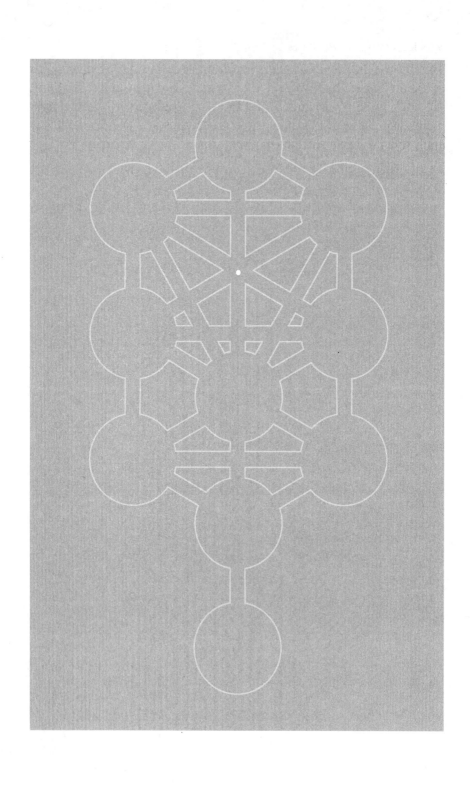

PHYSICAL METHODS

Notes on Healing

As Above, So Below

Listening to the Body

1
Notes on Healing

The information in this book is generally safe to use, however, each person must take responsibility for his or her own actions. If you have medical or psychological problems, then you must take care when using the modalities in this book. Find someone competent to integrate a healing program for you. Doing the balancing procedures should be helpful to almost anyone, but when you start moving energy in the body, be prepared for changes.

It is said that the nervous system and average human personality is unprepared to handle the full intensity of the spiritual current. It would be like plugging a 120 volt capacity wire into a 2000 volt outlet. I remember many years ago seeing a guru pass his energy to a girl, who immediately fell to the ground in a seizure. Her colleagues were pleased that her years of vegetarianism and meditation had finally paid off, thus providing her with an ecstatic trance. I also recall seeing her about five weeks later walking with a cane. She was rebuilding from the overload her nervous system had experienced.

I have had numerous experiences of going to breath workshops or meditation groups and being overstimulated, only to crash physically or emotionally a few days later. There are many ways to manipulate the body's chemistry or energy system to create a mind-altering effect. One is with mind-altering drugs, and another is through certain intense breathing techniques. This is not always a bad thing, but one must be careful. Twenty-five years ago, I realized that I was not prepared to do

16

certain extreme breathing techniques because of the negative effect they had on me. I was not ready. I learned that it was more important to build a stronger constitution and to deal with other issues before I took off on an accelerated "trip" with breath. (I am not talking here about the many safe breathing techniques used before and with meditation, or supervised by qualified teachers.)

I have seen many patients attend a seminar or training, undergo a new, intense therapy, only to have complications later on because it was too much for their current level of balance. This is common with austere diets. People sometimes read about a new diet or fasting program that promises great results and the diet seems logical to them. However, when they go on the diet, they find that they were not ready for it or that it was too strict for them. For instance, if a person lacks certain detoxification enzymes in the liver, then fasting might compound the problem by dumping more toxins into a liver that is already compromised. It is important to know where you are biochemically, psychologically, and physiologically when you start a new health program. This is especially true of exercise programs. Exercise is one of the best things we can do for our health, but if we overexercise or do not warm up and cool down and follow all the other rules that honor our unique individual physiology, then even exercise can be dangerous.

If a nerve does not receive adequate stimulation or have the proper nutrients it becomes weakened. When this occurs, the nerve becomes more sensitive to firing. According to a neurological concept called "transneural degeneration," if you overstimulate a nerve in this condition, it can result in its death. Unfortunately, many therapies, while appropriate in one situation, are too much in another, with the result being nerve death. The girl who received the guru's energy experienced this, as do many people getting therapies from well-intentioned physicians and healers. The bottom line is that we must be aware of where we are at any given moment in our homeostatic balance and must proceed from that point with proper respect. Each person must find his or her own unique balance; for one, that might be

17

fasting, and for the other that might be feasting daily on beef. There is no hurry, and no judgment.

When we experience the bliss or inner peace that often comes from deep meditation, it is also common to become aware of some pattern within the body or mind that needs attention. This may come immediately or some time later. It is a side benefit of meditation, not the purpose of it. For example, if you shine a light into a room that has not been cleaned in a long time, you will see things that need cleaning or rearranging. If you shine too much light in the room, it can be overwhelming to the cleaning crew. It is better for most people to clean and purify their inner rooms in a gradual way. Again, each person has his or her own limits to discover and honor.

The purpose of this discussion is not to scare anyone away, but to offer perspective on the healing (or spiritual awakening) process. Sometimes healing is instantaneous, but usually it is a long process with many steps and many levels of success and regression. The advantage of using the procedures in this book is that we will constantly monitor the body. When the body has had enough stimulation or change at one time, then no more circuits will test active. Take a break and continue at another time.

Some Thoughts on Nutrition

One major area not covered here is nutrition. This is a book about healing from a vibrational perspective, however, there are a few basic nutritional points to consider. It greatly diminishes the benefit of balancing the body if a person is on a bad diet and has glaring chemical imbalances. It may even be harmful. Many structural and energetic distortions are the result of a biochemical imbalance in the body. Therefore, I always begin with a biochemical evaluation when I work with a patient. It is essential that a person maintain a decent diet in order to experience optimal health. The problem is that we all have different nutritional needs. In applied kinesiology (see Chapter 3), we are able to assess a person's unique level and types of toxins, detoxification ability, neurotransmitter balance, and, to some degree, endocrine balance. We integrate the feedback of the body, patient history, and symptoms with standard laboratory data to arrive at a nutritional and life-style program for that patient. Again, it is always best to tailor the program to the client rather than to take it from the most recent best-seller.

However, there are a few guideposts that apply to most people. Most of us need more water than we are drinking and more vegetables than we are eating. In addition, none of us can digest trans fats (hydrogenated or partially hydrogenated fats), the kind you find in fried foods and almost all commercially processed food products. The body does not have enzymes to break down these dangerous fats. Further, we need to avoid the ubiquitous aspartame and other chemical additives. The level of pesticides and other chemicals in our foods is terrifying, and it is best to eat organically grown and locally harvested foods when possible. There are a thousand good (and 10,000 not so good) nutrition books out there, but it is enough to say that moderation and common sense (hard to find in the nutrition area) should suffice. We need water, vegetables, leafy greens, fruits, some quality protein, good nonhydrogenated oils, and moderation (which means we can occasionally have dessert!).

Systems That Modulate Change in the Body

The nervous system responds to all stimuli. The slightest thought, sound, odor, taste, mechanical movement, or touch sends a cascade of neural stimuli through the system to the brainstem and back. Therefore, whatever we do affects the nervous system. Similarly, anything we do also has a biochemical response. A nerve cannot activate without a corresponding biochemical reaction. Sodium, potassium, ATP, and neurotransmitter substances mobilize with the firing of a nerve. Endocrine glands secrete hormones in response to stimuli, and so on. Clairvoyants tell us that the auric field, the energy field that surrounds the body, is in constant flux. They say that the colors and shapes they see are continually moving and modulating according to our experiences. An EEG or EKG demonstrates constant fluctuating electromagnetic energy. Therefore, we can see that the body is in constant motion on many levels simultaneously. Our neurology, chemistry, and energy states are in perpetual motion.

We could describe a response to a stimulus from any one of these perspectives and be correct. In this work, we will challenge the strength of muscles to observe their responses to stimuli, but how you describe it is up to you. You could say that the body reacted, that the nervous system reacted, that the energy system reacted, or that the body chemistry changed because of the provocation. All of these terms are accurate and interchangeable.

The main stimuli that we will use are hand signs called mudras, Hebrew and Sanskrit words, and touching areas on the body. Hand mudras are specific arrangements of the fingers and hands that have meaning to both the nervous system and the consciousness. These cause activation of the Kabbalah pathways, leading to stimulation in the nervous system, in the biochemistry of the body, and a change or movement in the energy systems that envelop the body. The mudras in this book function to awaken and stimulate different areas of consciousness. They form a Sign Language of the Soul. Therefore, a clairvoyant would be able to see a change in the energetic system, or auric field, whereas the applied kinesiologist would demonstrate the response via a muscle test. The body is a unified, coherent, integrated whole. We cannot affect one area without affecting all other areas as well. Therefore, we will use the terms nervous system, body, and energetic system interchangeably.

The Triad and Tetrad of Health

The "Triad of Health" (Figure 1.1) is a popular model for discussing the multiple aspects of healing. Applied kinesiologists often use this triangle as a way of describing the many approaches they incorporate into their therapy. The symbol is an equilateral triangle, with the base of the triangle representing structural health, one side representing biochemical health, and the third side representing psychological or energetic health. Structure relates to posture, spinal alignment, and body mechanics.

20

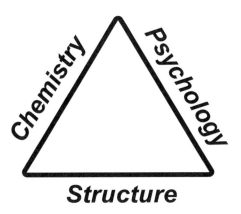

Structure

Figure 1.1 The Triad of Health

All of the manual therapies are included here, chiropractic, massage, craniosacral therapy, osteopathy, orthopedics. Chemistry relates to nutrition, allergy, toxicity, hormonal balance, and so on. The Psychology side of the triangle obviously relates to mental and emotional issues, but also includes energetic therapies, such as acupuncture, breath work, magnetic therapy, Therapeutic Touch, Polarity Therapy, and Reiki. Many conditions that present as mechanical problems, such as low back pain, are often a manifestation of a nutritional imbalance. Many biochemically related problems, such as blood-sugar irregularities, are often rooted in the psychological side of the triangle. A person can feel quite irritable when a headache results from a neck misalignment, and many low-back problems in women are hormonally related. Therefore, it is important to consider all three sides of the triad of health when seeking the cause of, and remedy for, any condition. Moreover, treating any one side of the triangle affects them all. Therapies can only manipulate the structure, the biochemistry, or the psychology/energy system. Healing is up to the individual.

I would like to propose that the triangle is not just a two-dimensional figure, but needs to be three-dimensional. The simplest three-dimensional object is the tetrahedron. Adding a point above the center of the triangle to represent the spiritual dimension of health, results in a tetrahedron (Figure 1.2). Interestingly, one of the more important hand mudras that we will discuss is in the shape of a tetrahedron.

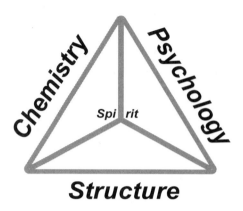

Figure 1.2 The Tetrad of Health

It is not popular in most traditional health arenas to talk about spiritual health or the spiritual perspective. One reason may be that such discussion often digresses into a religious, dogmatic, or proprietary perspective. The exceptions are in the areas of pastoral counseling and end-of-life care for the terminally ill. Furthermore, we all think that our own view of the heavens is the correct one. And this is rightly so. Each of us experiences a unique connection to the divine. The problems come when we interact with others and are unable to honor their unique spiritual connection. In any case, the model of health cannot be complete unless we acknowledge the spiritual dimension in each individual. The goal here is not to convince the person of some new way of thinking; the spiritual point of the tetrahedron of health is a focal point for interacting with the other three sides of the base triangle. Addressing the structure, chemistry, or psychology with the spiritual design in mind allows a greater chance for a positive outcome. Good healers always come from this perspective of the tip of the tetrahedron, because they have love and concern for their clients. Love is the nature of spiritual reality, and no other philosophy or technique is necessary beyond that. However, using the hand signs to center the body to the deeper levels of the soul can give this love a better chance to flow in our patients and in ourselves.

The Attitude of the Healer

This book focuses on protocols and procedures designed to align the body-mind to the higher patterns of the Tree of Life. However, that is not enough. There is no substitute for sitting with another person with compassion, patience, love, and without judgment. This quiet internal space is necessary for any healer, therapist, or friend to develop. Perfecting this ability negates the need for anything in this book! It is important to understand that people can experience a certain health condition for a variety of reasons, some of which may, or may not, be of their own doing. We must be in the space of seeing another person as part of a larger life system, with forces operating on him or her that are beyond our comprehension and so should be beyond our judgment.

It is essential, therefore, that you apply these balancing procedures to yourself first. This work requires balance, centeredness, humility, patience, sensitivity, and focus. I hope these methods will help you to become a better healer or therapist, and also will help you with your individual needs. The important thing to remember, however, is that we do not heal others. We are gardeners cleaning out the weeds and caring for the plants, and so on, but we do not cause the plants to grow. There is great danger in this work or any powerful approach if you allow your ego to think it can control spiritual forces. The Kabbalah is a system of explaining infinite reality, however the intellect alone cannot grasp it. It requires a major opening of the heart. The procedures in this book allow the therapist to follow the movement of energy through many levels of consciousness to a healing conclusion. There is no manipulation involved, because as soon as the procedures start, the body-mind-soul is always in control. Each step in these procedures follows the previous one. Therefore, the client is always running the show. All we do as therapists is follow the energy according to our understanding of its flow. We can feel good about the outcome, but we must always realize that the other person already has the pattern of healing within and that our part is small in comparison with that of the client's life force.

Please reread the previous paragraph.

2
As Above, So Below

One of the major tenets of the Kabbalah is that man/woman is created in the image of a greater Cosmic or Divine Being. The Hermetic aphorism "as above, so below" perfectly reflects this. If this is the case, then we should be able to see the cosmic design in our human form. In addition to our form's reflecting the higher pattern, our innate qualities of being are the same as those of the divine, as one drop of water has the properties of the ocean.

Eastern Philosophy

Let us first look at a philosophical and healing system in which the link between man/woman and nature has been well established. Eastern cosmology relates this in great detail. The duality of yin and yang, along with the interaction of five basic elements (fire, earth, metal, water, and wood), can describe everything in existence.

Yin, yang, and the five elements (Figure 2.1) build and destroy each other in such ways as to keep balance and health in the body-mind-spirit. Eastern medical philosophy relates every aspect of the body and every aspect of life to one or more combinations of these polarities and the five elements. There is a direct correlation with the elements of nature and their effect on the energies of the body. Each season relates to one of the five elements, and, as a result, that element is likewise stimulated in the human body.

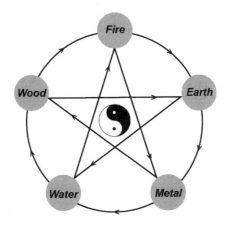

Figure 2.1 Five Elements

For instance, springtime relates to the element wood, and the liver is the organ connected to the wood element (Table 2.1). Often, people who have problems with their livers have allergies that worsen in the spring. Eastern medicine views man/woman as a part of nature and the greater cosmic life. We are a microcosm of the elements and meridians of nature.

Yoga

The yogis of India have a rich system of mysticism that uses the body as a tool for spiritual evolution. There are yoga postures, breath techniques, hand mudras, and many other physical methods of relating their cosmology to the body. The Tantric form of Hinduism delves most deeply into this area.

"According to Tantric principles, all that exists in the universe must also exist in the individual body. If we can analyze one human being, we shall be able to analyze the entire universe, because it is believed that all is built on the same plane. The

25

Element	Yang Organ	Yin Organ	Emotion	Taste	Voice	Season
Fire	Small Intestine	Heart	Joy	Bitter	Laughs	Summer
Earth	Stomach	Spleen	Sympathy	Sweet	Sings	Late Summer
Metal	Large Intestine	Lungs	Grief	Pungent	Weeps	Autumn
Water	Urinary bladder	Kidneys	Fear	Salty	Groans	Winter
Wood	Gallbladder	Liver	Anger	Sour	Shouts	Spring

Table 2.1 Element Correspondences

purpose is to search for the whole truth within, so that one may realize one's inner self, unfolding the basic reality of the universe." [2]

Kabbalah

The Kabbalah also correlates the macrocosm with the microcosm.

"So God created man in His own image, in the image of God created He him; male and female He created them." [3]

Therefore, Kabbalistic images often relate to the human body. This is more than the anthropomorphizing of spiritual concepts; it is the relating of analogous structures between God and human. The relationship between our body and the cosmic design is the subject of this chapter although we will learn much more about the importance of the following numbers and images in later chapters. Then it will cease to be just a curiosity or coincidence, but will point the way to a practical approach to healing.

---

[2] Mookerjee, Ajit (1982). *Kundalini, The Arousal of the Inner Energy.* Rochester, VT: Destiny Books.
[3] Genesis 1:27

Hebrew	English	Cranial Bone	Hebrew	English	Cranial Bone
א	Alef	Occiput	ל	Lamed	Left palatine
ב	Beyt	Left temporal	מ	Mem	Left inferior concha
ג	Gimel	Right maxilla	נ	Nun	Right nasal
ד	Daleth	Right lacrimal	ס	Samek	Left zygomatic
ה	Heh	Frontal	ע	Ayin	Right palatine
ו	Vav	Right parietal	פ	Pey	Left lacrimal
ז	Zayin	Left nasal	צ	Tzadik	Left maxilla
ח	Chet	Right zygomatic	ק	Qoof	Ethmoid
ט	Tet	Right inferior concha	ר	Resh	Vomer
י	Yod	Mandible	ש	Shin	Sphenoid
כ	Caph	Left parietal	ת	Tau	Right temporal

Table 2.2 Correlation of Letter Pathways with Cranial Bones

4

The number 4 is the cornerstone of the Kabbalah. The Tree of Life manifests through four different worlds or dimensions. These four worlds reflect in the body through the four extremities. Just as there are two upper and two lower worlds, there are two upper and two lower extremities. The palms of the hands and soles of the feet are indicators of these four worlds. In addition, the heart chakra comprises four Sefiroth (see Chapter 10 for a discussion of the Sefiroth). These four Sefiroth parallel the four chambers of the human heart. There are also four letters in the Divine Name, YHVH, יהוה .

4 + 1

In addition to the four worlds of the Tree of Life, we must consider the roots of the Tree. Highest divinity "exists" in the roots. It is not a place, nor a state, but it just Is. The head in the body and the thumb in the hand symbolically represent the roots. The four fingers are somewhat similar, but the thumb is in a different plane and it is shorter than the fingers. The four extremities are somewhat similar, but the head is different. This is a parallel to the four worlds and the roots of the Tree.

10

*"Ten Sefiroth of Nothingness in the
number of ten fingers, five opposite five."* [4]

The 10 fingers (toes) represent the 10 Sefiroth. There are also 10 openings in the body. Seven are in the head (two eyes, two nostrils, two ears, and the mouth), plus the anus, the penis/vulva, and the umbilicus (closed at birth).

22

The number 22 is a special number in the Kabbalah. Twenty-two pathways on the Tree of Life connect the various Sefiroth. These pathways correspond with the letters in the Hebrew alphabet. The Sefer Yetzirah correlates each Hebrew letter with a different part of the body. Also, there are 22 individual bones in the skull. Table 2.2 shows the correlations derived from testing the resonances between the cranial bones and the pathways. Chapter 7 will explain how to do this testing.

The building blocks of proteins are the amino acids, the product of the DNA code. There are 20 of these and they are found in all biological systems. In addition to the amino acids, there are two punctuation marks in the DNA code that act as stop signals. Actually, there are three punctuation marks, but one is also an amino acid. The 20 amino acids and two stop codes of DNA correlate exactly with the 22 letters of the Hebrew alphabet. Table 2.3 gives the correlations of the amino acids with the Hebrew letters that have been verified to resonate in the body.

---

[4] Kaplan, Aryeh (1990). *Sefer Yetzirah, The Book of Creation.* York Beach, ME: Samuel Weiser.

Hebrew	Hebrew Transliteration	English Equivalents	Amino Acid
א	Alef	Alef	Stop
ב	Beyt	B	Valine
ג	Gimel	G	Isoleucine
ד	Daleth	D	Proline
ה	Heh	H	Tyrosine
ו	Vav	V	Cysteine
ז	Zayin	Z	Serine
ח	Chet	Khet	Asparagine
ט	Tet	Tet	Threonine
י	Yod	J	Aspartic acid
כ	Caph	C	Phenylalanine
ל	Lamed	L	Arginine
מ	Mem	M	Stop
נ	Nun	N	Histidine
ס	Samek	Sahm	Glutamic acid
ע	Ayin	I	Lysine
פ	Pey	P	Leucine
צ	Tzadik	TZah	Glutamine
ק	Qoof	Q	Glycine
ר	Resh	R	Tryptophan
ש	Shin	S	Methionine
ת	Tau	T	Alanine

Table 2.3 Amino Acids and Letter Pathways

29

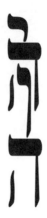

Figure 2.2 Vertical YHVH Showing Image of Man

26

Five of the 33 embryonic spinal segments eventually fuse together to form the sacrum, and four segments fuse to become the coccyx. This leaves the spine with 26 individual bones:

7 cervical vertebrae   12 thoracic vertebrae
5 lumbar vertebrae   Sacrum Coccyx

There are also 26 acupuncture meridians, when we include both sides and the midline meridians. The number 26 is one of the most important in the Kabbalah, as it is the numerical value of the Tetragrammaton, the four-letter name of God, יהוה, YHVH (Y=10, H=5, V=6, H=5). In addition, it is the sum of the numbers of the four central Sefiroth of the Tree of Life (1+6+9+10=26). Therefore, the sum of the central column Sefiroth, which resides over the spine, equals the number of bones in the spine. We will spend more time on this in a later chapter, but if you look at Figure 2.2, you will see that the vertical representation of the four-letter Name of God creates a human shape with a head, spine, arms, and legs. Truly, "God made man/woman in His/Her own image."

32

The 32 pathways on the Tree of Life consist of the 10 Sefiroth and the 22 gates or pathways that connect them. In the human body, there are 32 bones in each extremity. Table 2.4 shows the correlations derived from testing the resonance between the bones and the pathways. There are also 32 teeth in the adult mouth. This Tree is a very special one.

33

The spine represents the central column of the Tree. Powerful energy centers reside in the spinal system. The embryonic spine consists of 33 segments. Adding the nonmanifest "roots of the Tree" to the other 32 pathways gives us the full 33.

Kabbalistic literature is replete with diagrams of the Tree of Life superimposed on the body, the hands in various mudras, and Hebrew letters on the face, hands, and torso. Much of biblical imagery relates to the body.

> *"Tantrikas regard the human organism as a capsule of the whole. 'He who realizes the truth of the body can then come to know the truth of the universe' (Ratnasara). The adept accepts this with an almost existential awareness. The psychic and physical organisms are interdependent, since each makes the other possible. The forces governing the cosmos on the macro-level govern the individual on the micro-level. Life is one, and all its forms are interrelated in a vastly complicated but inseparable whole. The underlying unity becomes a bridge between the microcosm and the macrocosm."* [5]

The foregoing quote from a book on Tantra could just as easily be from a book on the Kabbalah or Chinese medicine. We develop great

---

[5] Mookerjee, Ajit (1982). *Kundalini, The Arousal of the Inner Energy.* Rochester, VT: Destiny Books.

Pathway	Upper Extremity	Lower Extremity
Kether	Scaphoid	Calcaneus
Hokhmah	Trapezium	1st cuneiform
Binah	Lunate	Talus
Hesed	Trapezoid	Cuboid
Gevurah	Triquetral	3rd cuneiform
Tifereth	Capitate	Navicular
Netzach	Pisiform	Ilium
Hod	Hamate	2nd cuneiform
Yesod	Ulna	Fibula
Malkuth	Radius	Tibia
Alef	Thumb distal	Great toe distal
Beyt	Clavicle	Pubis
Gimel	Scapula	Ischium
Daleth	Ring proximal	4th toe proximal
Heh	2nd metacarpal	2nd metatarsal
Vav	Little proximal	5th toe proximal
Zayin	Middle middle	3rd toe middle
Chet	Ring distal	4th toe distal
Tet	4th metacarpal	4th metatarsal
Yod	Humerus	Femur
Caph	Index middle	2nd toe middle
Lamed	Thumb proximal	Great toe proximal
Mem	3rd metacarpal	3rd metatarsal
Nun	Middle distal	3rd toe distal
Samek	5th metacarpal	5th metatarsal
Ayin	Little distal	5th toe distal
Pey	Index proximal	2nd toe proximal
Tzadik	Index distal	2nd toe distal
Qoof	Middle proximal	3rd toe proximal
Resh	Ring middle	4th toe middle
Shin	Little middle	5th toe middle
Tau	1st metacarpal	1st metatarsal

Table 2.4 Correlation of the 32 Pathways with the Extremity Bones

32

respect for the human form and the consciousness that inhabits it when we realize that we directly reflect the patterns that exist in nature, the cosmos, and the most Holy realms. The Kabbalistic patterns provide us with a road map to investigate the spiritual design in the human body. The map has been around for a long time and the physical correlations are well known. The exciting part, however, is our ability to navigate the spiritual map in the body. Through manual muscle testing, we will be able to see which of the many pathways is active or open for processing at any given time. In this way, the wisdom of the body, the inner being, or the nervous system (whichever you prefer), guides the balancing, centering, healing activity.

Margaret

Margaret, a 66-year-old woman, tripped and fell, injuring her right wrist, shoulder, and neck. She had no fractures or ligament damage but was still in considerable pain. After taking a history and doing an exam, I performed a gentle manipulation to the tendon in her right shoulder. Although this gave her shoulder considerable relief, it did nothing for her neck, wrist, and general soreness. Then I began the Sign Language of the Soul procedures. I centered and balanced her to the Tree of Life. After 7 corrections, the Tree of Life would no longer activate in the body. She felt overall improvement; however, there was still stiffness in her neck and wrist. Then I had her turn her neck to elicit the greatest amount of stiffness. With her neck in this position, I was again able to activate and balance her body to the Tree of Life. I had her continue to put her neck and wrist into positions that created discomfort, while at the same time activating the Tree of Life pattern. I also had her visualize the fall. In this way, I was able to apply the balancing methods to the specific areas of pain and distortion that were not "volunteering" for help. Eight more balancing sequences and she was almost pain free. The entire session took only 20 minutes.

3
Listening to the Body

The following discussion on applied kinesiology lays the groundwork for the simple technique you will learn later in this chapter. The work in this book, however, is not applied kinesiology. Applied kinesiology is a scientifically based analysis system that belongs in professional hands and is quite different from the many "kinesiologies" that fill the marketplace. I still use applied kinesiology techniques in my practice and could not function without them, and there is ample scientific research to support the basis of the muscle test and many of the procedures in applied kinesiology. However, the Kabbalistic-based procedures that I am presenting in this book are the product of my own observations and applications over many years. Although they have grown out of many treatment approaches and theories, they should not be confused with them. I have tried to remain grounded in the development of these methods, but it is up to you to evaluate their effectiveness on your own.

Applied Kinesiology

Applied kinesiology is a method of directly evaluating the body to ascertain balance or imbalance in any system. In 1964, George Goodheart, D.C., made the initial observations that led to the development of applied kinesiology. Standard manual muscle-testing procedures, or kinesiology, have been known for years. Pushing with resistance against a muscle will show either a state of strength or a state of weakness. Dr. Goodheart discovered that muscle testing could be applied in such a way as to allow the practitioner to learn more about the body than whether the muscle was just "strong or weak." This knowledge became known as applied kinesiology. Goodheart and his colleagues found correlations between many existing systems of therapy and the functions of muscles. For instance, Chapman's lymphatic reflexes correlate with the different muscles, and when the appropriate reflex is stimulated, it can have a beneficial or strengthening effect on a specific "weak" muscle. Each major muscle relates to a specific vascular reflex, spinal segment or nerve root, acupuncture meridian, nutrient, and organ. Since 1964, the literature of applied kinesiology and the scientific research that supports it has grown to make this one of the preeminent healing systems in the world.

In the last 15 years, there has been much research on the neurology of the muscle test. Muscle testing is a valid, objective assessment tool, and when correlated with other findings (patient history, physical exam, blood tests, x-rays), has great value in patient care. Muscle testing is a tremendous tool for evaluating neurological function. It can be very useful in evaluating the biochemistry of the body. Even the psychological side of the triad of health is amenable to evaluation by having a person vocalize certain phrases or visualize certain images and observe what happens in a muscle test. There are excellent, well-developed systems in all of these areas that have come from the years of research, both scientific and practical, by members of the International College of Applied Kinesiology (ICAK-USA).[6]

Kinesiology

Many lay healers have taken some principles from applied kinesiology and used them to develop or promote their own systems of healing. Some, of course, are much better than others are. Some people have used the muscle test with children regarding their education, and other areas not focused on in applied kinesiology. Occasionally, the muscle test is just a marketing tool to help sell a product. The problem with some of these muscle-testing methods is that there is no quality control.

---

[6] www.icakusa.com

The best muscle-testing procedures available to the lay public are taught by Touch for Health,[7] the organization that Dr. John Thie formed in the early 1970s and featured in his book by the same name. The basic muscle-testing procedures taught in Touch for Health have helped people all over the world. People who have a basis in this type of testing should have no trouble with the Sign Language of the Soul balancing procedures. If you want to learn more about muscle testing, you should read Dr. Thie's book.

Caveats on Muscle Testing

Many books teach self muscle testing with the fingers or the arm pull-down test. These methods can be highly unreliable. I have been muscle testing myself for over 20 years, and most of the observations in this book come from that testing. I can tell you, however, from vast personal experience that there are many pitfalls when you ask a biased person for information, and we are biased about ourselves. Early on, I made some almost disastrous mistakes when I believed what I tested on myself. I learned that self-testing was highly suspect, and I developed many checks and balances to evaluate the information I was getting. I also learned to rely on help from others when necessary. It is essential to have objective input as well as input from those further along the path than we are. A muscle test is just a piece of data, and nothing more. You cannot make a definitive statement about a person on the basis of a few muscle tests unless you have corroborating information. This is why the ICAK states that manual muscle testing needs corroboration by other data, such as a physical exam, patient history, x-rays, and lab work. You cannot diagnose cancer and other diseases with muscle testing, a point that is not taken into account in some of the lay healing techniques taught in weekend workshops. In addition, you cannot muscle test and ask who is going to win a horse race or where you should go to lunch today. Some people might be able

---

[7] Thie, John F. (1979). *Touch for Health,* Los Angeles, CA: DeVorss & Company. www.touch4health.com.

to do this, but they would be just as successful with a pendulum or tarot cards. This is getting into the psychic area. If you are already psychic, you do not need to use muscle testing.

The purpose of all this is not to scare you away from muscle testing, but to give a clear description of the strengths and weaknesses of this approach. Muscle testing is not a reliable method of diagnosis on its own, and it is not totally reliable in the hands of a novice. Research has evaluated the consistency of muscle testing among different examiners.[8, 9] Several muscle testers would individually challenge specific muscle groups in a patient with the results recorded. There was a high degree of consistency among those with five or more years of experience, but there was diminished consistency among those who had been working for less than five years. Clearly, taking a weekend course or only occasionally testing a person is not sufficient to develop reliable skills.

To recap and be clear about what we are going to do, let me restate that the procedures that follow are not applied kinesiology, or even Touch for Health. We will not be making diagnoses or giving physical treatments in this work. This approach is entirely reflex and vibrational in nature. You are going to learn a simple muscle test, as a feedback mechanism, in order to test the Kabbalah pathways. The goal is to learn how to read the body's response to a stimulus. There are many very advanced ways of reading the body, and it would be best to have some knowledge of them, but for this work, you just need to be able to observe a change in the state of a muscle. This indicates that there has been a change in the state of the nervous system because of some stimulus.

[8] Lawson, A., Calderon, L., Interexaminer Agreement for Applied Kinesiology Manual Muscle Testing, *Perceptual and Motor Skills*. 1997; 84:539-546.
[9] Scopp, Alfred L., An Experimental Evaluation of Kinesiology and Allergy and Deficiency Disease Diagnosis, *Journal of Orthomolecular Psychiatry*, Vol. VII, No. 2 (1978).

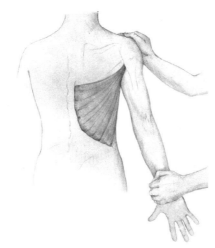

Figure 3.1 Testing the Latissimus Dorsi Muscle

A Simple Window Into the Body

Despite all the caveats about muscle testing, if we remain focused and do not take ourselves too seriously, we can gain a lot of information, even as beginners. We will challenge the strength of a muscle to observe the state of the body before and after a specific stimulus. The example we will use is the latissimus dorsi muscle. This muscle originates from a sheath at the side of the lower six thoracic vertebrae and is inserted at the back of the humerus near the shoulder (Figure 3.1).

You will need a partner for this procedure. Have your partner (sitting, standing, or lying) straighten one arm by his or her side with the elbow locked and the arm rotated so that the palm faces backward. It is important that the elbow remain locked and that the palm stay rotated backward. Your partner can "cheat" or override the test by bending the elbow or rotating the palm inward. As the tester, you stand beside your partner. You attempt to pull the arm away from the body by pulling it just above the wrist. The other hand stabilizes the body by resting on the same shoulder. Tell your partner to resist your pressure as you attempt to pull the arm away from his or her body. Do not overpower your partner, but pull firmly and confidently while feeling your partner's ability to respond. Remember that this is a test, not a

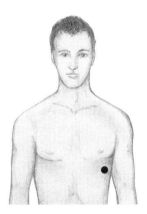 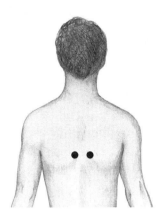

Figure 3.2 Neurolymphatics for the Latissimus Dorsi Muscle

contest. It is important that you monitor your partner's ability to lock the arm in place. You can ascertain the relative strength or weakness of the muscle in the first inch or two of the test. You do not need to be dramatic. Either the arm locks in place, or it does not. There is a tendency for the person to bend the elbow or rotate the arm if he or she senses that the muscle is weak. As the tester, you need to be aware of this. If the muscle does not test strong, test the other side in the hope of finding a strong muscle with which to work.

Occasionally, both sides will test weak. In that case, you have several options. Often the body is neurologically disorganized or confused, which results in incorrect readings, especially at the beginning of a session. There may be other reasons too, but there are too many possibilities to cover here.

This muscle shares a common nerve, lymph, acupuncture, and blood supply with the pancreas. Therefore, a weakness in this muscle might indicate a problem in this system, but it might not. There are other factors to consider before determining whether or not there is a weakness in the pancreatic system. It may be nothing more than the fact that the person is dehydrated or has not eaten recently. Therefore, if the muscle tests weak on both sides, you might have your partner drink

39

some water or eat some protein or carbohydrate, and then recheck the muscle. However, the person might need a chiropractic adjustment to the spine. You could also rub the Chapman's reflexes shown in Figure 3.2. These places will be sore if involved, and gentle massage might restore strength to the latissimus dorsi muscles. It is beyond the scope of this book to teach all the factors that can balance muscles. In this case, we are only attempting to find a strong muscle so that we can use it as an indicator for the effects of the procedures found in the later chapters.

If none of these procedures work, other biochemical or neurological problems exist that will require special attention. It is also possible to use another muscle for testing, if you have that knowledge. Performing the Tree of Life activation several times may also help to strengthen the muscle.

Assuming that the muscle locked in place and appeared to be "strong," you can now use it as an "indicator muscle." This muscle indicates a state of strength. In order to observe a change in the state of the muscle, have your partner utter a false statement aloud, such as, "My name is Sigmund Freud." As soon as he or she repeats this statement, retest the latissimus dorsi muscle. The muscle no longer should lock upon testing and it should appear weak. Do not panic if it does not test weak, however, because there might be other factors involved. Right now, we are just calibrating our tools and learning how to listen to the body. Now have your partner say, "My name is (real name)," and observe that the muscle now locks and appears to be strong.

When the arm does not lock, the muscle "appears" weak, but in actuality, there was no change in its strength. There was only a change in the state of the muscle. In neurological terminology, the muscle is facilitated when strong and inhibited when weak. Muscles get strong with exercise and weak with disuse, therefore, we will use the term inhibited to indicate when the muscle appears weak and facilitated when the muscle appears strong.

One advantage of using the hand signs and procedures taught

40

here is that when we apply a hand mudra or say a special Hebrew or Sanskrit word, we are focusing the body in a specific way. By focusing the body to a certain frequency or energetic state, we are telling the system that we want certain information; therefore, we are less likely to be led astray by existing disorganization in the body. Using the mudras alleviates many of the problems with accuracy encountered in muscle testing, because they focus the body on the inner patterns. This level is not subject to the same distortions encountered in a horizontal approach to health, meaning looking at the body as just a physical system. Just as in the universe, there is also a hierarchy in the nervous system. When we ask the central authority a question, we usually get a more accurate response than when we turn to a lower source. Focusing the body with one of the mudras tunes us to a higher level and allows us to rise above many of the compensations in the body. The deeper you can center the body, the less confusion you will encounter. The Tree of Life centering method taught in Chapters 12-16 removes all distortion from the system.

For now, experiment with some muscle tests and observe the response. There is no right or wrong answer. A muscle test can only show inhibition or facilitation, nothing more. Assuming that the latissimus test you did earlier appeared strong, or facilitated, use some other stimuli to see what happens. Have your partner touch an area on his or her body that is painful and retest the muscle. Have the person think of a painful memory and then a happy one. Observe the muscle response each time. Place a vitamin tablet (open a capsule) on the tongue to see whether it facilitates or inhibits the muscle. Do not make a judgment about the supplement on the basis of the muscle test. It may test weak or strong only at this time of day. Place an aspirin on the tongue and test the muscle. Stand in front of a TV set or pick up a cell phone and observe various responses to the testing. Play with it, but do not take any of your findings too seriously until you have more experience. Something is not necessarily bad for you because it weakens or inhibits a muscle. Learn to avoid making snap judgments or major decisions on the basis of a muscle test.

In the procedures in this book, muscles may inhibit when applying a hand mudra or using a Hebrew or Sanskrit word. In this case, it just means that there is a change or response to the stimulus in the body. If we place a mudra in the hands of the client and there is no change in any of the indicators, then we know that mudra had no appreciable effect on the system. If, however, the mudra triggers a change in the muscle state, we know that the body responded to the mudra. This is a positive response.

Chapter 7 will give you many opportunities to develop your skills. Manual muscle testing allows you to see how the hand signs resonate to the parts of the body, and the sounds of the Hebrew letters. This is how you will learn the mudras and their correlations. In addition, you will get practice observing the changes that take place in the body through the window of muscle testing.

Other Options

If you know muscle-testing procedures, you can use any intact muscle for the procedures in this book. Use a deltoid, quadriceps, or gluteus medius muscle if you wish. Since we will be using the mudras or words as filters, any intact muscle will do.

The best way to learn these procedures is to work with a partner. However, it is also possible to learn to feel the effect of the mudras within your own system. Place a mudra in your hands and observe your own inner reaction to it. If you correlate your inner feelings with the feedback of muscle testing, you can learn to calibrate your own sensing ability. This can take some time to learn, and one has to be careful not to let one's own ideas, or desires, take precedence over one's sensing, but it is possible. In time, you can become aware of the effect of the mudras in your clients as well.

It is not essential to use muscle testing to do the Tree of Life activation. However, it is quite helpful to follow the changes in the body as you apply the hand signs.

Finally, it is also possible to check leg lengths before and after a stimulus to the body. Any reaction to a stimulus will cause a visual change in the length of the legs from even to uneven, or vice versa.

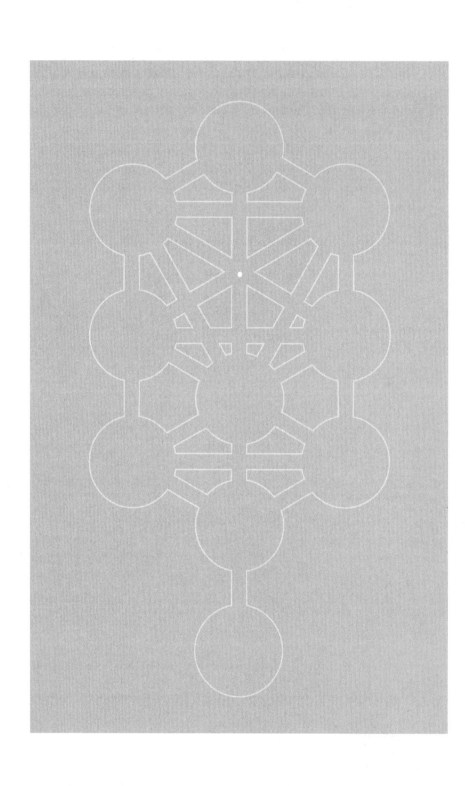

TOOLS

Hand Signs

The Shin Mudras

Language

Resonance

The term mudra, which comes from the root mud, means to rejoice. The Tantric tradition considers mudras to be "seals." They are used to seal, or lock into the body, certain energies or states of consciousness.

4
Hand Signs

"The hand speaks to the brain as surely as the brain speaks to the hand."

Robertson Davies, *What's Bred in the Bone*

The uniqueness of the human race lies in its language ability and the use of the hands, two functions that are tightly integrated. The hand has been a source of communication from the beginning of time. Most of us would find it very difficult to talk without using our hands. For the hearing impaired, hand signs are the voice of their language. We express emotion and the many subtleties of communication with gestures. We place our hands together to pray. With our hands, we can relate things that are impossible to express through the spoken word alone. Hand signals help us communicate to a person who is out of range of hearing, or when discretion is important. Aristotle considered the hands to be the "organ of organs, the instrument of instruments."

The language centers of the brain are situated primarily in the left hemisphere; however, it must be emphasized that a function as complex as language is wired into many other parts of the brain as well. Nevertheless, the left hemisphere is the dominant anchor for language, and this seems to be the case for any kind of language. Research has determined that sign language is neurologically facilitated by the same left-brain (mostly) locations as spoken language. Lesions in the brain that result in aphasia, loss of speech ability, also result in loss of signing in the hearing impaired.[10]

The development of gestures precedes that of vocalization. The child points at what he or she wants long before the child has the ability to ask for it. The use of the hand at least aids, if it does not cause, the development of language.

> *"The freeing of the human forelimb from its locomotor functions, and the consequent development of manipulative skills, is as important for the evolution of language as it clearly is for the evolution of technology."* [11]

Neurologist Frank R. Wilson, who wrote *The Hand*, theorizes that the hand played a major role in the evolution of language and that the movements of the hand and upper extremities helped to develop the language centers in the brain.

> *"... a gestural basis for the deep structure of language would have profound implications for cognitive science…because it would forge a powerful conceptual link between gesture and praxis, and compel consideration of the possibility that these two manual functions are critically linked in the brain itself."* [12]

In reviewing the work of anthropologist Gordon Hewes,[13] Wilson states:

> *"Early hominid tool use and the evolution of hemispheric specialization associated with hand use provide both the behavioral and neurologic context to account for the evolution of language."* [14]

---

[10] Wilson, Frank R. (1998). *The Hand*, New York: Pantheon Books.
[11] Place, Ullin T (2000). *The Role of the Hand in the Evolution of Language*. Psycoloquy: 11(007) Language Gesture (1).
[12] Wilson, Frank R. (1998). *The Hand*, New York: Pantheon Books.
[13] Hewes, Gordon, W. A History of the Study of Language Origins and the Gestural Primacy Hypothesis, in
Handbook of Human Symbolic Evolution, Lock and Peters, Eds.
[14] *Op. cit.*

Finally, he points out:

"Self-generated movement is the foundation of thought and willed action, the underlying mechanism by which the physical and psychological coordinates of the self come into being. For humans, the hand has a special role and status in the organization of movement and in the evolution of human cognition."

Thus, gesture is an innate human experience that not only precedes language, but also might be responsible for its development. A study of 12 blind individuals gives further credence to this theory.

"We found that all 12 blind speakers gestured as they spoke, despite the fact that they had never seen gesture. The blind group gestured at a rate not reliably different from the sighted group and conveyed the same information using the same range of gesture forms.... Blind speakers apparently do not require experience receiving gestures before spontaneously producing gestures of their own."[15]

It is no surprise then that the design of the nervous system relates information to and from the hands. The hands, along with the mouth and face, have a disproportionate amount of representation in the cerebral cortex. Figure 4.1 of the homunculus demonstrates that fact. Homunculus means "little man," and we can see from the diagram of the little man spread over the human cortex that the hands command a very large share of the cortex space, both motor and sensory. Wilder Penfield and Theodore Rasmussen, two Canadian neurosurgeons, published these findings of their research on the human brain in their 1950 book, *The Cerebral Cortex of Man*. Human evolution obviously required that the hands be central to survival, and this is evidenced in the amount of neural focus given them.

---

[15] Iverson, Jana, & Goldin-Meadow, Susan (1998). "Why People Gesture When They Speak," Nature.

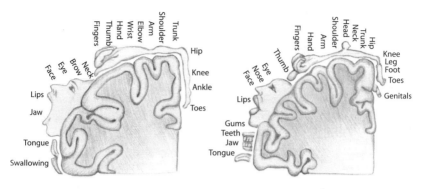

Figure 4.1 The Homunculus (From Cerebral Cortex of Man, by Penfield and Rasmussen,
Macmillan Library Reference, © 1950 Macmillan Library Reference.
Adapted by permission of the Gale Group.)

Hands in Healing

The use of hands in healing dates back to ancient times. The hands were the first healing tools. Laying on of hands, Therapeutic Touch, Polarity Therapy, massage, physical therapy, chiropractic, osteopathy, and surgery all require the skilled use of hands. The words chiropractic and surgery (chiurgia) both contain the root chiro, which is Greek for hands. The use of hands in energetic healing is beginning to be validated by modern research into biomagnetic fields.

> *"Medical research is demonstrating that devices producing pulsing magnetic fields of particular frequencies can stimulate the healing of a variety of tissues. Therapists from various schools of energy medicine can project, from their hands, fields with similar frequencies and intensities. Research documenting that these different approaches are efficacious is mutually validating. Medical research and hands-on therapies are confirming each other. The common denominator is the pulsating magnetic field, which is called a biomagnetic field when it emanates from the hands of a therapist."* [16]

---

[16] Oschman, James L. (2000). *Energy Medicine.* New York: Churchill Livingstone.

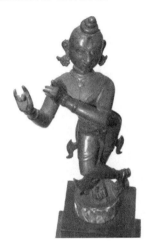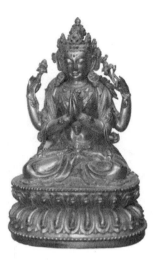

Figure 4.2 Statues of the Buddha[17]

The balance of this book is devoted to exploring ways to direct the specific frequencies that come from the hands by changing the configuration of the fingers and placing the hands in various positions.

Hand Mudras

The use of specialized hand signals called mudras dates back thousands of years. The term mudra, which comes from the root mud, means to rejoice. The Tantric tradition considers mudras to be "seals." They are used to seal, or lock into the body, certain energies or states of consciousness. Although they can refer to body postures as well as to specific hand signals, in this text, we focus only on the hands. The Polynesians use special hand positions in their dance rituals. They are used as a non-verbal narrative tool that expresses the story they are telling. The folklore beings of many Asian cultures are depicted with different mudras in their hands. Mudras are also prevalent in the hands of many Asian religious masters, and in images of their deities. Statues

---

[17] Thanks to Carmen Woidich and Carolyn Hatt for the Buddhas.

51

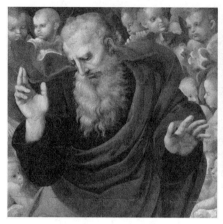 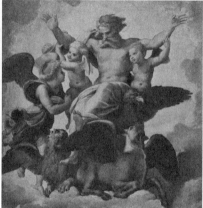

Figure 4.3 God   Figure 4.4 Vision of Ezekiel

and paintings of the Buddha show his hands in different mudras, and these mudras are still in use in Buddhism (Figure 4.2).

Likewise, statues of Hindu deities show different mudras in their hands. Practitioners of yoga use mudras to focus energy in certain ways during the postures (asanas), and especially during meditation. Each mudra has a mantra or Sanskrit power phrase associated with it, and the two often function together. We have all seen the thumbtips touching the index fingertips in people who are meditating.

There are many paintings and engravings depicting God, Yeshuah (Jesus), angels, saints, and other biblical personalities with their hands showing specific mudras. The paintings by Raphael[18] shown in Figures 4.3 and 4.4 depict specific hand mudras that we will explore in later chapters.

Kabbalistic literature includes many diagrams of the hands with Hebrew letters on the different joints, and modern rabbis continue to use the blessing mudra of the Levite priests (Figure 4.5). You will find many of these mudras in this book. Stan Tenen of the Meru Foundation

---

[18] Photographic Source: Archivi Alinari-Giraudon, Firenze

has done extensive research into hand positions relating to the Hebrew letters. You will find a lot of very interesting information on their website (www.Meru.org).

The ancient masters, saints, and teachers were communicating a message with their hands. These hand positions were not random, as they tell us something about the message or perspective of the teacher. It is not uncommon for people in deep meditation to have their hands unconsciously form specific mudras. The hands can, and do, reflect deep inner states of consciousness.

Clinical Kinesiology

Alan Beardall, D.C., one of the original applied kinesiologists, made many great contributions to the collective knowledge of the subject. One of his many accomplishments was the development of the therapeutic system that he called "Clinical Kinesiology." Central to this integrative approach to natural healing was the use of hand mudras. He called them hand modes. He once observed a patient spontaneously make a specific hand sign that altered the response of the muscle he was testing. This led him to research different hand positions and their effect on the body. He could ascertain the meaning of the different hand positions through manual muscle testing, observation, and a deep intuitive ability. Beardall developed several hundred of these hand modes that represented all parts and functions of the body.

For instance, the hand mode for a subluxation (a misalignment of a vertebra in the spine) is placing the side of the thumb against the side of the little finger at the last joint (Figure 4.6). If a patient places this mudra in one hand and it inhibits a strong muscle, it indicates that there is a subluxation somewhere in the spine. It is then possible to continue muscle testing while touching down the spine to find which vertebra counteracts this inhibition. This is the vertebra that needs correction. If the hand mode does not inhibit a muscle test, it is still possible to touch down the spine and to continue testing the strong muscle until touching one vertebra inhibits the muscle. Touching the vertebra without the hand mode might not inhibit

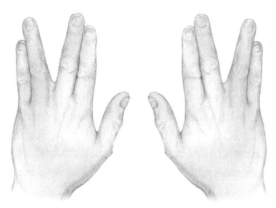

Figure 4.5 Levitical Blessing Mudra

a muscle and so not reveal the underlying problem. The hand mode acts as a neurological filter or focus point for the body. This is like sorting a list of names by the first name or the last name or the city the people come from, depending on the filter you have chosen. Beardall's hand modes enable the practitioner to get specific information from the nervous system. They help to give context to a dialog that you are having with the body. It is the difference between asking a general question and asking a specific one. This is a great tool for getting to deeper layers of distortion and imbalance in the body. With this technique, a doctor could literally "ask" the body where the problem lay, and if it needed acupuncture, nutrition, or a spinal adjustment to correct it.

There was some controversy in applied kinesiology surrounding the use of hand mudras. Some thought the mudras were mental concepts and did not really do anything in the nervous system. Those who used the mudras, however, found them to be a great aid to working with patients. It gave them a way to hold in-depth conversations with the body and to take their therapy to a new level. One common procedure used in applied kinesiology is to place the body in different positions when testing muscles. Some muscles will only exhibit inhibition (appear weak) when the patient is sitting, standing, or assuming the position of the original injury. It makes sense, therefore, to include specific hand

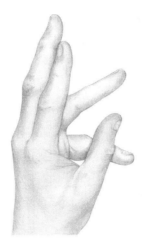

Figure 4.6 Subluxation Hand Mode

positions in muscle-testing procedures when we realize how much of our cortex is wired to and from the hands. We communicate so much with our hands that harnessing this tool can be a way to enhance our conscious dialog with the body.

The Master Circuit

Many years ago, I realized that I could muscle test myself (see caveats to doing this in the previous chapter). I could place the mudras in my hands and determine their effect on my body. I would spend some time each day doing very subtle balancing of my system as preparation for meditation. I was continually monitoring my feelings and awareness of my body to find where I needed balance. In the process, I developed many new balancing approaches to equate what I could feel within myself and what I could actually test with muscle testing and hand mudras.

In October 1983, at the end of a period of deep inner contemplation and work with some new modes that Beardall had just developed, I had a life transforming experience. My hands spontaneously went together in a hand sign that I had never seen before (Figure 4.7). I said

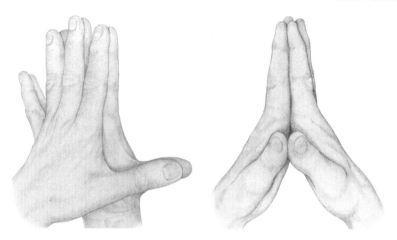

Figure 4.7 Two views of the "Master Circuit."

to myself, "I wonder what this means." There was an instantaneous reply. I heard a loud voice say, "This is the Master Circuit!" The voice came from all sides of me. I was stunned. Not one to hear voices, this was a memorable experience, because it was definitely not my little brain speaking to me. Furthermore, the effect of the mudra lasted in me for hours. Without going into more detail, this hand sign worked in my system like nothing I had ever experienced. It took approximately 13 years before I fully realized that it was the mudra for the Sefirah Yesod (Figure 4.8).

This mudra, which was my key to the Master Circuit, was the first of many hand signs given to me in my inner contemplations over the years. The mudra was active over only certain areas of my body, and the design of the active areas was quite different from anything I had ever seen. Soon after receiving the Master Circuit mudra, I recalled having purchased a book on the Kabbalah several years earlier. I did not think much of the book, or the Kabbalah, at that time, but I did remember the diagram of the Tree of Life. I retrieved the book and found that the new mudra was active over the locations of the 10 Sefiroth, the major energy centers of the Tree of Life (see Figure 10.4, page 111). This was the beginning of my research into the Kabbalah and how it is used to activate the spiritual patterns in the body. Since then, I have spent much time contemplating the mudras and the energies of the Tree of Life.

One of the characteristics of the Kabbalah is that the Tree of Life design, as the universal hologram, is present in every particle of creation. Every cell in the body contains the entire Tree. Therefore, as I was initially climbing my Jacob's ladder, it was like opening those Russian nesting dolls. You open a doll and find another inside, and another inside that one, and so on. Each new insight would cause the reflection of the 32 paths of the Tree to shift a bit in the body. The sequence of the mudras would change or the way the patterns were displayed in the body would shift.

Early on, I had only a limited number of mudras with which to work, but something was definitely happening with the ones I had. They were not enough, however, so I kept meditating, working on myself, and searching for new insights. Some mudras took over a decade to understand, some almost two decades. To this day, I continue to gain a deeper understanding of how it all fits together. I have no illusion that this system of healing is complete, as I frequently receive new insights about this work. Often I would spend months seemingly bogged down in what I thought was futile, only to find that I was being shown a completely new perspective. It was like climbing a ladder backward. You can see where you have been, but not where you are going. I gradually gained confidence that there would always be another rung to climb. Slowly, but surely, an unseen force guided me to each new level. Each level is but a subset of a greater level, but all the levels look the same. The anatomy of the Tree of Life, which we will discuss later, is always the same whether we are discussing quantum physics, the function of the liver, or the meaning of Genesis.

Spiritual masters or teachers use mudras to express the state of consciousness they are in or as a method of transferring that energy state to others. In our case, we will use the mudras as inputs to tune the body to these different states. We will also use them to tune others to these energy states. The hands can communicate to both the external world and the inner awareness. If the inner awareness can use the mudra to make a shift, we will observe this fact by a change in the state of a muscle. Our ability to test the body's response to a mudra will tell us where we can, and cannot, go with this work. This will keep us working in cooperation with the Inner Being, which is connected to our nervous system "until death do us part."

One unique aspect of these hand mudras is that they generate a frequency state that remains in the body until another specific focus comes along. The effect of Dr. Beardall's hand modes lasts as long as they are in the hands. The hand mudras in this book generate a state in the body that persists until another focus becomes dominant. In other words, if you open your hands after placing one of the Kabbalah hand signs, the body will remain tuned to that frequency. If you put in a new mudra, speak, or mentally focus on something else, the effect of the mudra releases. This will be useful to us later when we start to test how the hand mudras resonate to words, biochemical substances, and body points. The mudra can be placed in the hands and then released, and for a time the body continues to respond as if it were still in the hands.

Alternatives to the Hand Mudras

The hand mudras presented here are all fairly easy to make, although they will be easier for some people than for others. I hope that you will find them interesting and experiment with them to gain experience. This work grew out of using these hand signs and evaluating their effect on the body. However, it is important to emphasize that it is not necessary to use the hand mudras to do the balancing procedures described in this book. There are several alternative methods for activating the Kabbalistic patterns in the body. For instance, each hand mudra correlates with a specific Hebrew or Sanskrit word. Many of the mudras correlate with specific places you can touch on the body. If you find the mudras confusing or difficult, do not despair. You do not need to be a finger contortionist to learn these methods.

58

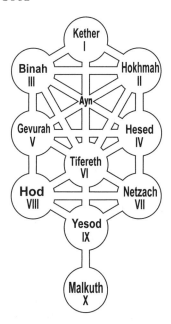

Figure 4.8 Tree of Life

Looking at the pictures of the mudras works as well as placing them into the hands. If you have difficulty making a certain mudra and you are unsure of how to pronounce its corresponding word, then just look at the picture of it. This will have the same effect as if you had placed the mudra in your own hands.

Respect for the Mudras

Although I initially learned the hand mudras through research into my own system, I soon found that when they worked in me, they would also work in everyone else. The hand mudras presented here focus the nervous system on different energetic levels or states of awareness. Most of these levels are beyond normal waking consciousness, although the hand signs themselves do not necessarily cause a conscious shift in consciousness. They cause the body or nervous system to resonate, for a moment, to that level. If you have the sensitivity and are able

59

to shift your state of awareness, then the mudras will take you there. For most of us, they just cause the physical system to resonate to that consciousness so that a healing process can occur. However, you must understand that working with the hand signs and the centering procedures will cause changes. You might feel spacey or suddenly hungry as you experiment with them. Do not be surprised if emotional issues begin to surface or if new insights come to you as the result of placing your fingers in different positions. The mudras are powerful, especially when used with the proper visual focal and when used at the right time. Therefore, anyone with psychological or physical problems, or anyone using mind-altering drugs or psychoactive medications, must not use these methods without supervision by a qualified therapist.

With all of this in mind, I would ask those who use or study the mudras, to honor them as sacred symbols of states of awareness that we strive to achieve within ourselves. They are a Sign Language of the Soul. Therefore, it would be inappropriate to wave these mudras about in public. Be discreet when working on others. It is best to have the client focus on the healing instead of on the modality of the healing. It is not necessary that your client see the mudras for the effects to occur. In fact, it is not necessary to use the mudras at all, as we will see. There are substitute methods that are easier and faster for most people. The mudras are not a secret, but it would be inappropriate to expose them in certain settings. The best attitude to take is to respect and honor them as indicators of sacred and holy vibratory states, and to act accordingly.

Ella

Ella, a 28 year old woman, had been experiencing low back pain since a fall while skiing two months earlier. An exam revealed only biomechanical misalignments, subluxations, and muscle imbalances. I performed only the Sign Language of the Soul procedures. Five such attunements corrected almost all of her problems. Then I had her get into a position that still caused her some discomfort (squatting) and quickly activated the Tree of Life once more. She was back to normal with no hint of any discomfort in her body. Ah, the joy of youth!

5
The Shin Mudras

The 21st letter of the Hebrew alphabet is the Shin. This letter looks like a W (ש) and is equivalent to the "sh" or "s" sound. The Shin is one of the three "mother" letters, together with Alef and Mem. The mother letters relate to the elements, with Shin representing fire, Alef representing air, and Mem for water. In the numbering system of the Hebrew language, the Shin is the symbol for 300. The *Zohar* calls it "the letter of truth." [19] Shin is "mythically considered to be the 'spirit' or 'breath' of God; in fact, the organic process of cosmic life." [20] The letter is in the shape of a tooth, so that is a correlate for this letter, and it also corresponds to the head. On the Tree of Life, Shin is the gate between Hesed and Gevurah at the shoulders. The Shin correlates with the amino acid methionine.

This letter consists of three upright "heads." There are numerous interpretations of the meaning of these heads, some positive and some negative.[21] On the negative side, they relate to "jealousy, uncontrolled appetite, and desire for honor." [22] On the positive side, they reflect the three aspects of soul: Nefesh, Ruach, and Neshamah (see Chapter 12). Taking it out of the personal realm, we could also relate them to the gross, subtle, and causal worlds.

---

[19] *Zohar*, Benei Yissaschar, Part One, 75b.
[20] Suares, Carlo (1968). *The Sepher Yetsira*. Boston: Shambhala.
[21] Munk, Michael L. (1983). *The Wisdom of the Hebrew Alphabet*. Brooklyn, NY: Mesorah Publications.
[22] Glazerson, Matityahu (1991). *Letters of Fire, Mystical Insights into the Hebrew Language*. Spring Valley, NY: Feldheim.

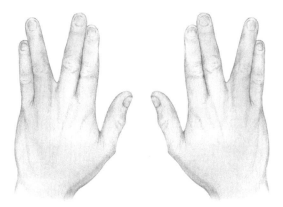

Figure 5.1 Levitical Blessing Mudra

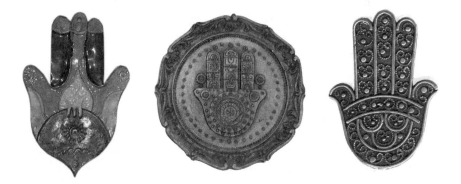

Figure 5.2 Hamsas

It is possible to create Shins in the hands by placing the fingers in specific positions, and thus the term "Shin mudras." The idea for these mudras came from several sources.

First, the blessing mudra of the Levite priest shows a three-headed Shin in each hand (Figure 5.1). This hand mudra had intrigued me for many years, but I was unable to understand this most important mudra until the rest of the mudras of the Tree were in place (see Chapter 15).

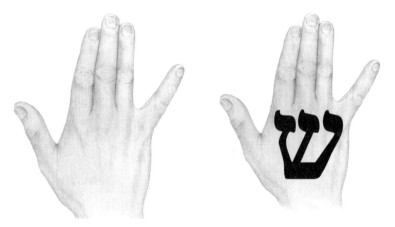

Figure 5.3 Hamsa in Hand   Figure 5.4 Shin on Hand

Second, on a trip to Israel years ago, I became fascinated with the abundance of hand symbols in the jewelry and art of the Middle East called hamsas (Figure 5.2). This is the name for hand in Hebrew, which literally means "five" as in the number of fingers on the hand. My interest in mudras led me to investigate this symbol of good luck and good fortune. By placing the index, middle, and ring fingers together and separating the thumb and little fingers, we get a mudra that looks like the hamsa. This hand sign (Figure 5.3) was ultimately found to relate to the brow chakra. This three-headed mudra resembles the letter Shin (Figure 5.4). It is possible to create five other Shins with the various finger combinations. Figure 5.6 shows the six Shin mudras.

Chakras

Chakra is a Sanskrit word meaning wheel. Chakras are vortex wheels that move energy from one state to another. There is much literature on the chakras, dating back to the Tantric Hindu tradition. Tantric philosophy describes these energy centers as focused areas of consciousness. They are psychic energy reservoirs that "govern the whole condition of being."[23] There are literally thousands of chakras,

---

[23] Mookerjee, Ajit (1982). *Kundalini, The Arousal of the Inner Energy*. Rochester, VT: Destiny Books.

Sanskrit	Chakra	Nervous System (Plexus)	Meridian	Neuro-transmitter	Endocrine	Sound
Sahasrara (violet)	Crown	Brain	CV/GV GV20 L&R	Dopamine	Pineal	(C) 540
Ajna (indigo)	Brow	Carotid	LU/LI	GABA/ glycine/taurine	Pituitary	(B) 480
Visuddha (blue)	Throat	Pharyngeal	TW/CX	Aspartate/ glutamate	Thyroid, parathyroid	(A) 432
Anahata (green)	Heart	Cardiac	HT/SI	Noradrenaline	Thymus	(G) 384
Manipura (yellow)	Solar plexus	Coeliac or solar	LV/GB	Acetylcholine	Adrenal	(F) 360
Svadhisthana (orange)	Sacral	Splenic	ST/SP	Histamine	Pancreas, spleen	(E) 324
Muladhara (red)	Root	Coccygeal	K/BL	Serotonin	Gonads	(D) 576

Table 5.1 Chakra Correspondences

but only six major chakras align with the spine. A seventh chakra, called the crown, which sits above the head, contains all the frequencies of the lower six (Figure 5.5). The chakras are not physical, but are located in the subtle energy fields. Clairvoyants and other sensitives are able to see or feel these energy vortices and to describe them in great detail. Even though the chakras are not tangible in the material sense, they do have physical associations. They relate to the neurological plexuses along the spine and to the major endocrine glands. Table 5.1 lays out just some of the many associations with the chakras.

For years, I had known that the six Shin mudras related to the six spinal chakras, left hand for the left side, and right for the right. However, what I eventually realized was that the chakras activate in a much deeper way in the body if a hexagram or six-pointed star is made with each pair of Shin mudras. These mudras focus the body on the frequencies of the chakras.

The three heads of the Shin of each hand give the six "points" of

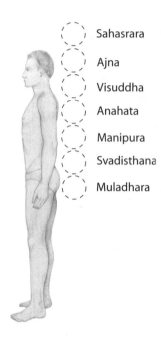

Sahasrara

Ajna

Visuddha

Anahata

Manipura

Svadisthana

Muladhara

Figure 5.5 Chakras

the star. Therefore, the hands can form six different six-pointed stars. The six star Shin mudras are shown in Figure 5.7. It is not necessary to rotate the hand 180 degrees for the mudra to work, as long as the palms touch and the fingers of the opposite hands do not align with each other.

Another, easier way to form some of the chakra mudras is to open the hands and cross the thumbs. However, this only works with the three chakra mudras in which the thumb is not adjacent to the index finger. Therefore, it is possible to make the Ajna, Anahata, and Muladhara mudras with the thumbs crossed. Visuddha, Manipura, and Svadisthana are not amenable to the open position because the thumbs engage the index fingers. Figures 5.8-5.10 show the open positions for the Ajna, Anahata, and Muladhara chakra mudras.

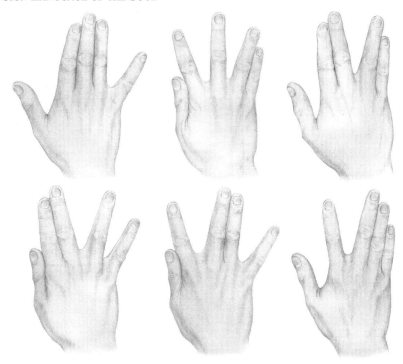

Figure 5.6 The Six Shin Mudras

6

The number 6 is very important in the Kabbalah. Six is the first perfect number. A perfect number is when the sum of the whole numbers that divide into it (except for itself) equal the number. For instance, 6 can be divided by 1, 2, and 3, which when added together equals 6 (1+2+3=1x2x3). Perfect numbers are rare. Between 0 and 1,000, there are only three perfect numbers (6, 28, and 496). The book of Genesis tells the story of the six days of creation. The main symbol of Judaism, the six-pointed star, is a symbol of these six days.[24]

The first word of the book of Genesis is B'reshith, בראשית. These six letters are commonly translated as "In the beginning," but as many as

---

[24] Leet, Lenora (1999). *The Secret Doctrine of the Kabbalah* Chapter 6. Rochester, VT: Inner Traditions.

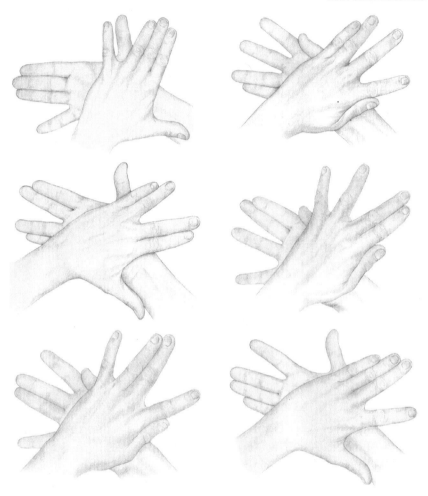

Figure 5.7 The Six Star Shin Mudras of the Chakras

70 different interpretations have been ascribed to these letters, depending on how they are subdivided.[25] The most popular alternative meaning is, "He created six" by splitting B'reshith into two smaller words that become, "He created" and "six," Bara Shith, שית ברא.[26] Therefore, we see that the first word of the book of Genesis describes the process of six, the

---

[25] *Tiqunim HaZohar*, 1558.
[26]Sperling and Simon, translators. *The Zohar,* p. 65. London: Soncino Press.

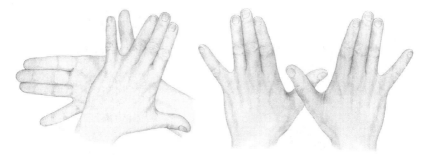

Figure 5.8 Equivalent Mudras for the Ajna Chakra

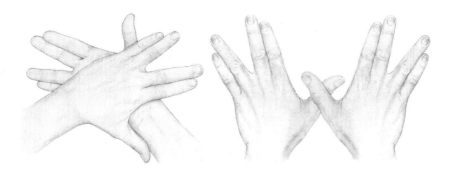

Figure 5.9 Equivalent Mudras for the Anahata Chakra

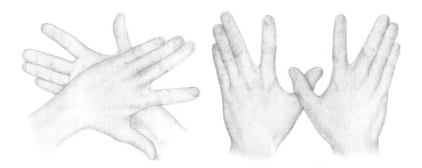

Figure 5.10 Equivalent Mudras for the Muladhara Chakra

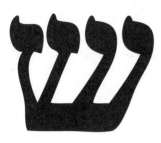

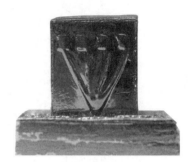

Figure 5.11 Quad Shin   Figure 5.12 Quad Shin on Tefillin

six days of creation. The importance of this first word of Genesis cannot be overstated.

The number of the Shin is 300, but two Shins give us 600, and dropping the zeros gives us 6. The perfect number 6 becomes the perfect set of mudras, of which only six possible hand combinations exist.

The Quad Shin Mudras

Most people who know Hebrew are familiar only with the typical three-headed Shin, ש. There is, however, a four-headed Shin, which can only be found on the Tefillin (Figure 5.11 and 5.12). Observant Jewish men use phylacteries as part of their prayer ritual. These consist of two separate small black boxes with scrolls inside. Attached to each box is a set of leather straps. One box goes on the left upper arm with the straps wrapped in a special way down the left arm and hand. In fact, a three-headed Shin is usually formed in the left palm by the manner in which the strap is wrapped. The other box, which contains four compartments, each with a scroll inside, goes on above the forehead. The four compartments of the Tefillin remind us of the four worlds of the Tree of Life. Interestingly, Orthodox Jews use the Tefillin six days a

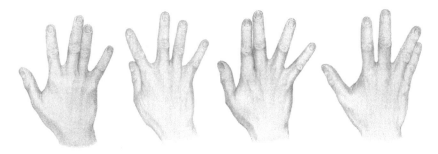

Figure 5.13 Quad Shin Mudras

week and approximately 300 days a year since they exempt the Sabbath and other holidays.[27] On the right side of the head Tefillin is a regular three-headed Shin. On the left side of this box is the four-headed Shin. It is a metaphysical letter in that the fourth head represents the world to come. As we shall see shortly, this quad Shin represents the four worlds of the Tree.

As you have probably figured out by now, it is also possible to make the quad Shin with the hands, and there are only four ways to do it (Figure 5.13).

These four mudras, each placed bilaterally, relate to the four worlds of the Tree and to the four nucleotide bases of the DNA. They also correlate exactly with the four-letter Name of God, YHVH, יהוה, (Yod, Heh, Vav, Heh) (Figures 5.14-5.17). Two different mudras resonate to the letter Heh, H, ה. The letter is the same, but the meaning of each is different, hence two mudras.

The main mudra, or the first one of the sequence, is that depicted on the hands of angels, saints and other spiritual teachers as seen in paintings and sculpture. This mudra is the most important of the four. This particular mudra resonates to the Hebrew letter Yod, י, in the Holy Name (Figure 5.14). The letter Yod can be used to make all the

[27] Kaplan, Aryeh (1974). *The Aryeh Kaplan Anthology, II*. Brooklyn, NY: Mesorah Publications.

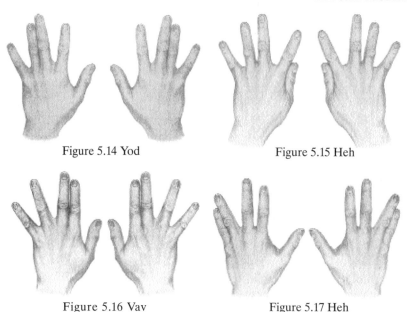

Figure 5.14 Yod   Figure 5.15 Heh

Figure 5.16 Vav   Figure 5.17 Heh

other letters and is the one with which the World-to-Come was created.[28] This statement bears itself out because this Yod mudra forms the basis for at least 8 other mudras.

Summary

We have seen that very simple finger positions act as filters to focus the body/nervous system/energy system on a new frequency. These mudras are organic in the sense that the fingers naturally generate all the combinations of four and six. There are no leftover mudras. These hand signs are the basis of much of what we do in this work. In actuality, the hand mudras are not necessary, since it is possible to substitute the corresponding words for them. The advantages of the hand signs is that they anchor the resonance directly to the body, they give us the opportunity to demonstrate the resonance between different methods of activating the Kabbalistic energies, and they are the basic tools to which we can always return as we climb the Tree of Life.

---

[28] Kaplan, Aryeh (1974). *The Aryeh Kaplan Anthology, II*. Brooklyn, NY: Mesorah Publications.

6
Language

"Language, as well as the faculty of speech, was the immediate gift of God."
Noah Webster: American Dictionary, 1828

"In his whole life, man achieves nothing so great and so wonderful as what he achieved when he learned to talk."
Ascribed to "a Danish philosopher" in Otto Jespersen,
Language, 1922.

Everything is language. If we had no language, we would have no world. With language, we can form relationships with our environment. Language is what ties us together. The development of the human psyche and of the human nervous system depends on language. There is a theory that left- or right-handedness is a product of language development. We all know about the body language that reveals our unsaid feelings. Applied kinesiologists and other body therapists understand a kind of body language that enables them to talk to the body to learn its needs.

There is also a language of movement, such as dance. Rudolf Steiner developed a system of movements based on language called Eurythmy, in which each sound or letter resonates to a special type of movement pattern.[29] We have a full alphabet of movements available

---

[29] Spock, Marjorie (1980). *Eurythmy.* Spring Valley, NY: The Anthroposophic Press.

to us. Curative Eurythmists study a patient to see which letters of movement are missing and they prescribe those movements as therapies. It is highly effective for many conditions, especially in children.

The Kabbalah gives us the Divine Language. It states that the universe is a constant emanation as an expression of 22 letters. The *Sefer Yetzirah* gives the scenario of letters and their meanings as they continually create the Word, which becomes the material universe. All books on the Kabbalah or other mystical teachings emphasize the power of language. In Hinduism, the word Om or Aum is the root word that is the sound of creation. Mantras or seed words are meditation tools used for their effect on centering the mind, awakening energy centers, and moving energy.

Hebrew, like Sanskrit, is a root language. Modern Hebrew and Sanskrit are different from their ancient versions, Sinatic Hebrew and Brahmi Sanskrit, and it is possible that both stem from an earlier common source. Still, these languages are special in that the sounds and symbols of the words, for the most part, relate directly to the Higher or Spiritual planes of existence. In other words, the sound of a word activates the energetic form of the material object referred to by the word. If you said the Hebrew word Yad, ד, it not only would refer to a hand, but also would call up the archetype of a hand. A good clairvoyant would be able to see the energy form of the hand even if he or she had not heard the word, because the person speaking the word would have generated the archetype with his or her voice. Languages today are representative and do not reflect the closeness to the inner worlds that the original languages did. Language has decayed from its closeness to its original source, as it is now more suited to today's materialistic culture than the ancient tongues would be. When we consider how slang, jive, rap, advertising, and other wordplay have altered the English language, we can see the distance we have moved from our Latin roots. Likewise, our language is even further away from its spiritual roots.

Certain words in Hebrew and Sanskrit have special meanings and the power to effect change. Chanting these words is said to create

74

powerful effects in the soul. In both of these languages, there are special names given to the divine, divine beings, or divine attributes. The purpose here is to discuss how to speak these power words, in both Hebrew and Sanskrit, in such a way that they have the maximum effect on the nervous system. And when we speak these words in the proper way, it has the same effect as using its corresponding hand mudra. This gives us two ways to activate the Kabbalistic patterns in the nervous system.

Orthodox Judaism teaches that, as a sign of respect, certain Hebrew names of God are not to be spoken aloud. "Thou shalt not take the Lord's Name in vain."[30] Only the High Priest of Israel could speak the Holy Name, on one day a year, Yom Kippur, and only inside the Holy Sanctuary of the Temple. In the same vein, Orthodox Jews will not write the name God unless they leave out the "o." Thus, if anything happens to destroy the page, the Name of G-d is not defaced. Many Jews take this practice quite seriously. Therefore, it is best if we also show respect for the sacredness of the hand mudras that equate to the Holy Names.

Four Doorways

The Tree of Life expresses through four worlds or dimensions and in the body there are four doorways that resonate to these worlds. These doorways are the area 2 to 3 inches below the navel, the heart, the third eye, and the upper neck. Focusing on one of these doorways tunes the body to that world. This will be greatly expanded upon in Chapter 9, however, the basic concept of the four doorways is important to the following discussion.

You can speak the Hebrew and Sanskrit worlds aloud, you can silently mouth them, or you can intentionally think them. No matter which method you use, it is essential that you concentrate on one of the four areas of the body that act as the doorways for the world. In other words, when you focus on these areas of your body the words are equivalent to the mudras.

---

[30] Exodus 20:7.

Let us take the mudra for Yod as an example. You can use the hand sign shown in Figure 5.14 or you can just say Yod (yood as in good) aloud. If you choose to think the word, then you must intentionally think the word as opposed to letting it idle in your mind. In this way, you are projecting the word with your mind, so it has an effect. The other way is to silently mouth the word. In the development of this work, all "spoken" words were silently mouthed as this bypassed the subconscious mind's filtering mechanism. There is actually a neurological basis behind this. However, after learning how to focus on the doorways to the four worlds, this became unnecessary. You need to focus your attention on one of the four doorways to the worlds, when speaking or thinking the name of the mudra, or when placing the mudra. All are equivalent in their effect. The advantage to speaking, mouthing, or even whispering is that you are using a physical method to create the frequency of the word. Thinking also works, but for some people, this might be more difficult. You need to consciously project your thought as an intention when you do this. I recommend that you use one of the other methods at first. By using your hands or voice you are activating the language centers of the brain to cause a resonance within the soul. This is the link between the heavens and the earth. It is interesting that the ancients considered the larynx, the voice box, to be a small uterus. They are similarly shaped and both are creative instruments that give life. Language was the tool that birthed the manifest universe and with our larynx we express our ideas and emotions. The uterus is the vehicle that births the child.

There is one final note worth mentioning regarding the neurological aspect. In Chapter 4 on hand signs, we saw that the homunculus showed that the hands were disproportionately represented in the cerebral cortex. The other area that was about equal in representation to the hands was the face, including the mouth. The face and mouth are the center of many functions, but the movement of the lips and tongue in speech and language can attest to a large part of this emphasis in the brain.

We now have the second tool for investigating the patterns of the Kabbalah in the nervous system or in the body. Hand mudras and their corresponding spoken words are equivalent. Touching certain points on the body also activates the Kabbalah pathways. There are biochemical equivalents, as well, although they are of no use in activating the pathways. Thus, there are many ways to activate the patterns once we have the map and the correlations between systems. Always remember that these pathways relate to cosmic, universal patterns. We are only working with physical analogs to the macrocosmic pattern. This universal pattern exists on all levels. The key is to be able to test when resonance with the higher pattern has occurred so that we can consciously follow the energies in the body in order to further balance and improve an individual's health.

Larry

Larry came into my office complaining of left lower back pain. It was worse with standing, sitting, and walking long distances. He appeared to have a typical misalignment of his sacroiliac joints and bottom lumbar vertebra. In addition, there were several dysfunctional pelvic muscles. He had seen several chiropractors for this condition, but it kept recurring. Although this was a typical chiropractic problem, I chose to center him to the Tree of Life using the Sign Language of the Soul methods. After 8 of the balancing procedures, which took less than 15 minutes, he was pain free. He later stated that he had longer term relief from this treatment than any of his previous forms of therapy. Sometimes the reason that the structure is unstable has deeper roots and in this case the Tree of Life balancing procedures were quite effective.

7
Resonance

"That which is above is like to that which is below, and that which is below is like to that which is above, to accomplish the miracles of the one thing." [31]

Understanding the concept of resonance is essential to this work. When a note is played on a guitar, a nearby string will begin to vibrate or resonate to it if the notes are similar. They may be of different octaves, but if the notes are the same, resonance will occur. Resonance is re-sounding. When another, yet different, vibration sounds again in a sympathetic manner, there is resonance. Another term for resonance is entrainment. This is a physics term used to describe what happens when two rhythms, which have nearly the same frequency, synchronize with each other. This occurs, for instance, when you have several pendulum clocks on the same wall. Eventually they will entrain and all swing at the same rhythm.

Resonance in the Body

In this work, we are exploring a cosmic map that reflects itself in many different ways in the body. All the maps are the same, 10 Sefiroth and 22 letter pathways, except that they are operating in different octaves or dimensions. Therefore, the pathway for Kether in one map

---

[31] Hermes Trismisgestis.

should resonate to a pathway for Kether in any other map. Resonance occurs any time you use two different methods to activate the same pathway. Whenever this type of resonance occurs in the body, it results in the inhibition of a strong muscle.

When we are attuned to the spiritual Tree of Life, our body and mind resonate to and reflect this state. The goal of all mystical systems, and, one hopes, all religions, is to realize oneness with the Spiritual Source. When the body and mind are aligned with the Higher Design, we feel whole on many levels. This is one reason why the procedures presented here have such a positive effect.

Resonance Between People

The other form of resonance or entrainment that we can observe occurs between two (or more) people. People who live and work together may find that their patterns begin to fall into rhythm with each other. Women who live together for a while often report that their menses occur at the same time. People who sit quietly together find that their breathing synchronizes. Listening to music or to a great lecture or story entrains the listeners to the rhythm of the music, words, or images. Many in the audience will exhibit similar physiological and emotional responses. This is why we like to be with happy, fun-loving, exciting people. We are resonators, and the longer we are with someone, the more we entrain ourselves to his or her rhythms. This is one reason why it is a unique learning experience to be in the presence of a spiritually realized master such as Ammachi, Mother Meera, or Sai Baba.

If a person has a Tree of Life pathway activated in his or her nervous system, it can affect someone nearby. In other words, when you place a Kabbalistic sign in your hands and stand near somebody else, the other person, if quiet and centered, will also resonate to the frequency of the mudra. The same holds true for saying the names of the pathways as long as the other person focuses on one of the four doorways. Therefore, if you activate a pathway with intent, a person near you will react to it. This way, you can work with other people without having them perform the mudras or pronounce the Hebrew words. This is much faster and more practical than teaching the mudras/words to each person. If the other person is not distracted, the activation of the pathway will maintain itself even after you remove the mudra from your hands, or after you have finished saying the name of the mudra.

If you think about it, we are always interacting with others on a vibrational basis. We can feel the emotional state of those near us, even without visual clues. Someone who is visually impaired can verify this. Even if we are not consciously aware of another person's attitudinal or emotional state, it still affects us if we are in proximity to him or her. Science has developed many ways to evaluate the electrical nature of the body, such as the electrocardiogram (EKG), electroencephalogram (EEG), and electromyogram (EMG). This same instrumentation has corroborated the affect we have on one another.

> *"There is evidence for coupling of both cardiac and brain rhythms between two individuals in the same room who are sitting quietly, facing each other, with eyes closed, without touching (Russek & Schwarz 1994, 1996). The electro-cardiograms and electroencephalograms of both individuals are recorded, and the rhythms are analysed for the presence of between-person cardiac-brain synchronization. Such synchronization is present..."* [32]

Newer instruments are able to measure the biomagnetic energy that emanates from different parts of the body. For example, recording devices, up to 15 feet away from the body, have detected the biomagnetic emanations of the heart. Furthermore, quantum physics shows us that the distance over which we can affect others may be infinite.

---

[32] Oschman, James (1997). What is Healing Energy? Part 2, *Journal of Bodywork and Movement Therapies*, 1(2), 117-128.

Seeing Is Believing

It is possible to validate the many correlations described in this book by using muscle testing. It is one thing to say that this system connects to this pathway, and so on. Many researchers have done this. It is quite another to demonstrate that they do, in fact, relate to each other. This chapter will show how to do this.

All you need is a basic understanding of muscle testing. Like any new skill, it takes practice to become good at these techniques. Remember that the results of muscle testing become more reliable as the tester becomes more experienced. However, you need to start somewhere, and testing these resonances can afford good practice. Just be patient if your results aren't yet completely accurate.

A Word of Caution

Performing the various tests offered in this book will help you understand what the mudras and words do in the body. It is important to be able to follow what is happening in the body as you tune it to the higher design. Our goal is to develop a therapeutic approach to help balance the body on the basis of these patterns. When running one of the balancing procedures, it is very important that all four worlds on the Tree be activated in the body. In the following examples, however, we will not be concerned about opening all levels of the Tree. If you feel spacey, or start to react to the movement of energies, stop and rest or get something to eat. If that is not enough, then activate the Tree of Life as described in the summary at the end of Chapter 16. Most people will not have any problem with these experiments, but if you do have a reaction, this should bring you back into balance. Do not do these exercises when hungry. The mudras/words require physical energy, and sometimes just eating a snack will alleviate any discomfort.

The following experiments will help you learn the concept of resonance and give you a chance to make some of the mudras and use their Hebrew words. The mudras are covered in later chapters, so do not concern yourself with their meaning or application at this time.

81

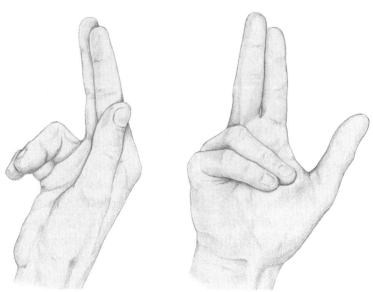

Figure 7.1 Two Views of Kether Mudra

The First Test: Kether

Find a partner with whom to work so that you can practice testing the resonance between the mudras, words, and body points. Always begin by checking your partner to see that you are starting with a facilitated latissimus muscle and that it inhibits when you have them state their incorrect name. Make sure that, as the tester, you are centered and objective. Review the procedures for muscle testing in Chapter 3. Now that you have calibrated your tools, it is time to perform an experiment.

Place the Kether mudra in your right hand. Just flex the ring and little fingers without touching them to the palm. Keep the index and middle fingers straight and close to each other or touching. The thumb is straight, but apart from the index finger (Figure 7.1).

You can leave this mudra in your hand since it requires only one

82

hand, or you can remove it just before testing. Test it both ways. You can also let your partner make the mudra. Place the mudra near your partner so that he or she will resonate to this frequency. Make sure that his or her latissimus dorsi muscle appears strong. Then have your partner concentrate on the area 2 to 3 inches below his or her navel while one of you says the word Kether (Keh tur). The area below the navel is the doorway to activate the lowest of the four worlds, Asiyah. This will become clear in Chapter 16. Challenge the strength of the muscle. If you have done everything correctly, the muscle will appear weak. (If it does not inhibit, see below.) The inhibition of the muscle should persist until you put in a new mudra, or your partner says another word, even if your partner stops concentrating on the area below his or her navel. Test to see how long it takes before the muscle returns to strength. Have your partner walk around and take some deep breaths. Ask him or her to say something or place a new mudra. Experiment with different activities to see what releases the body from the frequency of the mudra.

Now test it another way. Make sure that your partner is back in a facilitated state and the muscle appears strong. If the person is not, have him or her say something aloud to break the previous resonance. Place the Kether mudra in your hand again and now touch (either of you can do this) the top of his or her head (see Figure 10.5, page 112). Again, your partner must concentrate on the area several inches below his or her navel. To repeat, a muscle that appears weak upon testing indicates resonance. The muscle is not "weak"; it is in a state of inhibition for a moment. This "weakness" does not need correcting. It only means that the two things relate to each other. Weakness is a state of strength, but inhibition is a state of function. Here we are evaluating the function of the nervous system in response to various stimuli.

You should now see the resonance between the hand mudra, the word Kether, and the body location point of the first Sefirah, Kether. You should also have some idea about how long the effect of a mudra will last in the body. Do not forget to feel within yourself the connection between the mudra, its word, and its location point. All the correspondences in this book have been well tested, and should demonstrate resonance if properly applied. If there is no resonance, there are several things you can consider.

1. Reevaluate your muscle-testing technique. Make sure that you are centered, objective, and confident in your testing. It takes practice and experience to become proficient in a new endeavor. Remember that it is a test, not a fight. Learn to feel your partner's response to your attempt to pull his or her arm. Sometimes it is necessary to do a few of the balancing procedures on yourself before you become clear enough to test the resonance.

2. Be sure you do the hand mudra properly. It is possible to remove the mudra from your hands right after forming it as the effect of the mudra will last, but if you have problems, make sure to keep the correct mudra in your hands.

3. Be sure that your partner concentrates on the area below his or her navel, or one of the other doorways. The mudras do not generally activate unless there is a focus on the doorway to one of the four worlds. The doorway to the lowest world is located behind the area below the navel, which is called the Tan Tien. The other doorways are the heart, third eye, and the area at the base of the skull/top of the neck (see Chapter 9).

Resonance

This concept is so important to this work that it bears repeating. Resonance occurs between people as well as within the nervous system of an individual. In the latter case, resonance always occurs when you activate the same pathway in two different ways, or in two different dimensions. Saying the name resonates to its hand mudra, which resonates to its body location, which resonates to its biochemical substance, and so on. Resonance always causes a shift in the state of a muscle that is tested. Since we start with a facilitated muscle, the shift in state is always to inhibition (weakness). The state of the muscle will remain inhibited until a new focus is initiated in the nervous system. Although the muscle appears "weak," this does not indicate that something is wrong. Resonance does not mean an imbalance. It is merely the body's way of showing a shift in state because of the stimulus.

On the other hand, muscle inhibition during a balancing sequence indicates a positive mudra/word. Keep in mind that the mudras/words move energy or focus the nervous system to a different frequency. Placing a positive one, to which the body reacts, will cause a change to occur in the nervous system that results in muscle inhibition, but once the energy has moved and the nervous system has reset itself to the new frequency, the muscle inhibition will cease. It is as if the body goes into neutral while the system is shifting gears. While in neutral, the muscle appears weak, but it returns to a strong state as soon as the new "gear" or frequency engages. Therefore, it is necessary to perform the muscle challenge when initiating the mudra so as not to miss the possible response.

When demonstrating resonance by inputting two different stimuli for the same pathway, the inhibition will remain as long as there is no new stimulus or focus in the body-mind. The body does not change gears in this case. An internal change comes only when the body-mind is ready to move to the new level. This is the beauty of this system. Muscle testing enables us to navigate the many pathways to reach the desired destination. The inner wisdom determines the destination and the path to follow, not the intellect of the therapist or the client.

Feel It Yourself

The best way to demonstrate resonance is to feel the correlation between the various modalities within you. When you place your hands in a mudra, focus on the appropriate world, and then say or think its Hebrew word, you should be able to feel the resonant effect. This will become easier to do as you work with them. It will help to attune you to your own inner Tree of Life.

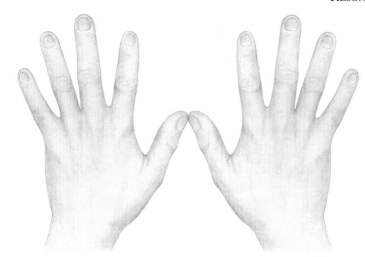

Figure 7.2 Binah

Binah

Experiment with the third Sefirah, Binah (Figure 7.2). The physical location of Binah is on the anterior surface of the left wrist (palm side) just proximal (toward the body) to the crease of the hand (Figure 10.6, page 112). The hand mudra is all fingers straight and apart with the tips of the thumbs touching. The thumb tip of one hand can overlap the thumbnail of the other hand, and is a bit easier to do than touching the tips of the thumbs. Either way is fine.

Make sure that your partner's latissimus dorsi muscle is facilitated (strong). Touch the left anterior wrist and then have your partner say the word Binah (bee nah). Then retest the latissimus dorsi muscle. Most likely there will be no resonance. Now, have your partner focus on the area 2 to 3 inches below his or her navel and repeat the word Binah. Test the latissimus dorsi muscle again. This time there should be inhibition, which indicates resonance. Place the mudra and then have your partner say the word Binah. Test the latissimus dorsi muscle again. There should be a resonance between the hand mudra or anterior wrist and the word Binah, causing an inhibition of the muscle. Test the muscle with all the dual combinations of the three different methods of

86

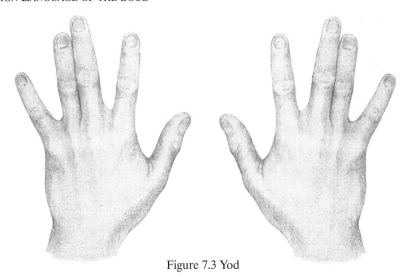

Figure 7.3 Yod

stimulating Binah to observe the resonance, but do not forget to focus on the area below the navel.

    left anterior wrist + mudra
    mudra + word Binah
    word Binah + left anterior wrist

Now, instead of saying the word Binah, think it, while holding the hand mudra. This should also resonate.

Yod

The Yod mudra resonates in all four worlds, which means that your partner can concentrate on any of the four doorways when you test for resonances. The doorways are located at the area 2 to 3 inches below the navel, the heart, the third eye (1/2 to 1 inch above the eyebrows), and the area at the base of the skull. Make sure that the latissimus dorsi muscle in your partner is facilitated (strong). Have your partner focus on one of the four doorways and then place and remove the mudra shown in Figure 7.3. It is not necessary to keep the mudra in your hands for more than a few seconds. Then have your partner say the word Yod (yood as in good) and challenge the latissimus dorsi to observe the change in its state. Remember that the effect of the mudra will last until you create another major focus in the nervous system. Therefore, it does not need to stay in your hands if your partner remains quiet. This word, in combination with the hand sign, will create resonance in the body. It should not matter whether you or your partner places the mudra or who speaks the word. Both of you will be resonating to the same frequency. Looking at Figure 7.3 is also equivalent to placing the mudra.

The mudra will resonate between worlds as well. Make sure your partner is back to a facilitated state. Now have your partner focus on his or her heart area while you place the Yod mudra. Then have your partner focus on his or her third eye while you maintain the mudra. Next retest the latissimus dorsi muscle, which should inhibit, since you have activated the same pathway in two different ways (worlds).

If you are sensitive, you will be able to feel in your system the resonant response between the mudra and the word. If you cannot feel it, do this experiment with a partner and verify the resonance with muscle testing. Check the other three quad Shin mudras for resonance to their respective letter names, Heh, Vav, and Heh (Figures 5.15-5.17).

What is most important to take away from this chapter is the concept that the nervous system can show us when we stimulate the same energy pathway in two different ways. A muscle challenge inhibits if the nervous system receives two different inputs that target the same area. This is how many of these correlations and procedures were developed, and it is how we can demonstrate, learn, and utilize them.

Ron

Ron learned how to do this work in order to help his wife who was undergoing chemotherapy. Although skeptical by nature, he managed to perform the Tree of Life activations by having her look at pictures of the mudras. Here are his comments.

'Angie had quite a bad reaction to her newest chemo and the doctor had her take a rather strong steroid to counteract the side effects. It worked, but it left her hyper, feeling bad, and unable to sleep. I did your procedure and within ten minutes she was asleep. She got through the night quite well.'

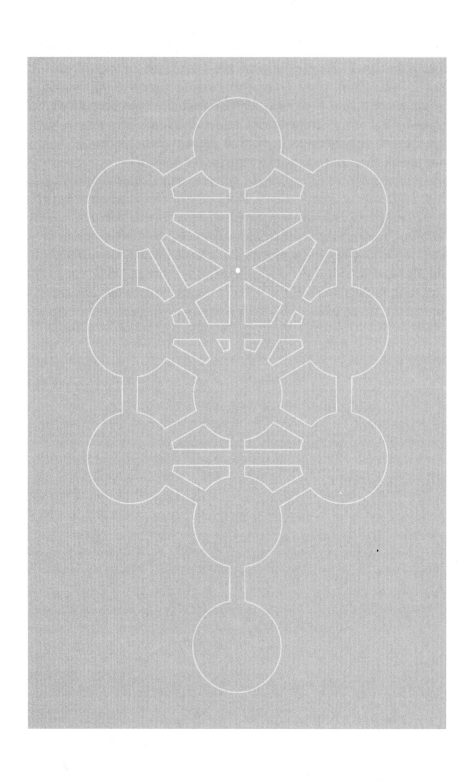

ANATOMY OF THE TREE OF LIFE

The Tree of Life

The Four Worlds

The 10 Sefiroth

The 22 Letters

"And in the midst of the Garden stands the Tree of Life, whose branches spread over all forms and trees and spices in fitting vessels. All the beasts of the field and all the fowls of the air shelter beneath the branches of this Tree. The fruit of the Tree gives life to all. It is everlasting. The 'other side' has no abode therein, but only the side of holiness. Blessed are they who taste thereof; they will live forever and ever, and it is they who are called 'the wise,' and they are vouchsafed life in this world as well as the world to come."[33]

[33] Sperling, Simon, & Levertoff, translators (1984). *The Zohar, Vol. III.* London, England: Soncino Press.

8
The Tree of Life

The Kabbalah teaches that God, HaShem, hollowed out a circle within Himself, and in that space, He created the universe. This first act of creation, called Tzimtzum, was the withdrawing or contracting to allow space for creation. Within this space followed the successive stages of creation. According to the Kabbalah, there are 10 phases in this creation process, which are repeated in each of four dimensions. Each dimension is denser than the preceding one, until the lowest one, which is the material plane. We image it as higher to lower, but in effect, it is only one system within the big circle of God. One image of the Tree of Life depicts a set of 40 concentric circles representing these 10 principles manifesting through the four dimensions or worlds, with the material universe in the center. It even looks like the cross section of a tree with its many rings.

The more common picture of the Tree of Life concentrates on one set of these 10 creative principles. It consists of a unique arrangement of 10 circles, called Sefiroth (Sefirah is singular), which literally means spheres. They are placed in three columns with three Sefiroth on each side and four in the central column. Twenty-two pathways, or gates, connect these 10 Sefiroth in a special relationship. These 22 pathways and 10 Sefiroth represent the 32 attributes of the Macrocosmic Being, called Adam Kadmon. This first Adam is the template from which man/woman was created and we saw in Chapter 2 how many times the numbers 4, 10, 22, and 32 appear in the body. The symbol of the Tree, as we will call it, is the cosmic blueprint, a holographic design of

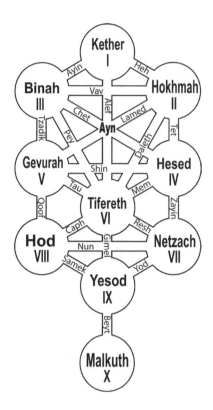

Figure 8.1 Tree of Life [36]

Creation. A hologram contains the entire information of the picture in all parts of itself. Cutting a holographic picture in half creates two complete pictures (although slightly diminished in quality). Every particle of the universe has this design in it, right down to our cellular level and into quantum physics.[34] Therefore, we can describe any human function with this model. All major world religious and philosophical systems fit the Tree pattern with its 10 circles connected by 22 lines.[35] We can use the design of the Tree to investigate anything. In this text,

---

[34] Leet, Lenora (1999). *The Secret Doctrine of the Kabbalah*, Chapter 9. Rochester, VT: Inner Traditions.

[35] Belk, Henry (1974). *A Cosmic Road Map and Guide Analysis*, Self-published.

[36] Adapted from: Feldman, Daniel (2001). *Qabalah, The Mystical Heritage of the Children of Abraham*. Santa Cruz, CA: Work of the Chariot.

we focus primarily on the body-mind, our personal copy of this cosmic system.

This symbol of the Tree did not appear in print until the 1600s, but there is evidence that it was known much earlier. The Kabbalah has a long oral tradition, so this knowledge was passed down verbally from generation to generation. There are linear, circular, and three-dimensional layouts of the 32 pathways. The different arrangements have been the source of much discussion in the many books about the Kabbalah. The Tree shown in this chapter is the fallen Tree, which manifests in Asiyah, the dimension of physical reality (Figure 8.1). As such, it aligns itself well with the human body. Another version is the Tree of Perfection, which also aligns to the body, but represents the nonfallen state of human consciousness (Figure 10.1).

Since the Kabbalah reveals hidden knowledge about creation, it is not surprising that the book of Genesis provides much imagery concerning the Tree of Life, and this is where we find its first mention.

> *"And out of the ground made the Lord God to grow every tree that is pleasant to the sight, and good for food; the tree of life also in the midst of the garden, and the tree of knowledge of good and evil."* [37]

Adam and Eve were forbidden to partake of the Tree of Knowledge of Good and Evil, but not the Tree of Life.

The *Sefer Yetzirah*, also called *The Book of Formation*, is one of the core Kabbalistic texts. It is deeply mystical, and many have pondered its message over the centuries. It describes how HaShem uses these 22 letters and 10 Sefiroth to create the universe, and as a text on the formation of the universe, it closely follows the book of Genesis. Aryeh Kaplan in his commentary on the *Sefer Yetzirah* states:

---

[37] Genesis 2:9.

"According to Kabbalists, these 32 paths are alluded to in the Torah by the 32 times that God's name Elohim appears in the account of creation in the first chapter of Genesis. In this account the expression 'God said' appears 10 times, and these are the Ten Sayings with which the world was created. These Ten Sayings parallel the Ten Sefiroth-The other 22 times that God's name appears in this account then parallel the 22 letters of the alphabet. The three times in which the expression 'God made' appears parallel the three Mothers. The seven repetitions of 'God saw' parallel the seven Doubles. The remaining 12 names parallel the 12 Elementals."[38]

Owing to the universality of the Kabbalah, many different people have been attracted to this study. They have added and subtracted components according to their own purposes and understanding. Christian mystics, occultists, and others have adopted portions of the Kabbalah into their own philosophies. Therefore, some diagrams of the Tree differ in the naming and numbering of the pathways. There are also differences in the correlations with the letter pathways, as the various schools of Kabbalistic thought differ in their perspective and purpose. There are always a multitude of approaches and interpretations in any field of thought, especially when the original concept is experiential in nature.

The Work of the Chariot version of the Tree, shown in Figure 8.1, with its letter pathways, stems from the *Sefer Yetzirah*, and it agrees with what the body shows with muscle testing. The charts and pathways from Feldman's book, *Qabalah, The Mystical Heritage of the Children of Abraham*, are ones that I have found to correlate with the body and that work. A search of Kabbalistic writings can become confusing and possibly overwhelming with all the information available. My purpose has been to use only what "works" and to test and retest it to ensure that it will work for others as well.

---

[38] Kaplan, Aryeh (1974). *Sefer Yetzirah, The Book of Creation*. York Beach, ME: Weiser.

The Roots of the Tree

It is important to keep in mind that while the Sefiroth represent the 10 stages of creation, they do not represent the Creator. It is possible to pay too much attention to the Sefiroth, the pathways, and the four worlds of the Tree of Life, and to overlook the roots of the Tree. The Tree of Life is an upside-down tree with the roots at the top. The Tree is manifest, and, therefore, observable. However, its roots are intangible. These roots are the Source of Life, and are considered to originate in a "negatively existent," pre-Will and premanifestation state. It is difficult to talk about negative existence, since it is a concept beyond our conscious understanding. Those who experience this state describe it by allegory and reference. When one reaches awareness of the negatively existent roots of the Tree, the material universe dissolves and only Oneness remains. It is beyond duality. The Hindus call this blissful state nirvikalpa samadhi and the Buddhists call it nirvana. The first commandment, "Thou shalt have no other Gods before me," [39] refers to this state.

The roots are collectively referred to as Ayn Sof. There are three roots to the Tree in this negative existence: Ayn, Ayn Sof, and Ayn Sof Or. Ayn (pronounced like "line") means Nothing, or Not. That which is Not is negative existence. Ayn Sof (pronounced like "sofa") means Limitless and Ayn Sof Or (pronounced like "oar") means Limitless Light. First Nothing, then Limitless, and then Limitless Light, and out of this the first Sefirah, Kether, is born. The meaning of these three symbols is beyond the scope of this work; it is the ultimate study and accomplishment of the mystic or religious adept.

---

[39] Exodus 20:3

Linda

Linda, a 38-year-old medical assistant, came to see me complaining of fatigue and gastric discomfort. In discussing what was going on in her life it became apparent that she often had these same problems when she was home visiting her family. Her childhood had been turbulent, leaving many scars. She related that, after being with her family there was often a drastic drop in her business in the following weeks. Clients would stop coming to see her and money would become scarce. It could take a month or more to recoup the loss in business flow. I performed several general attunements using the Sign Language of the Soul procedures as a base treatment. Then I had her visualize her business while at the same time inwardly giving honor to all her family members. This immediately caused a muscle test to appear weak. I applied the Tree of Life activation process again to help clear this pattern. It was interesting that her body showed great stress in the adrenal glands and the stomach area after the visualization. She needed to repeat the visualization approximately 10 times before the pattern was clear. She felt much calmer and even looked younger once the deep stress was relieved. Two days later I received a call from Linda stating that she had gone to a casino with her family and that she had won $2000! Not only that, but, two new clients had left messages on her office phone seeking appointments. All this occurred while she was still with her family. Now, not all cases of lack of abundance will clear this easily, but Linda had a particularly dramatic turn-around, which demonstrates the potential use of these procedures.

9
The Four Worlds

The Tree of Life with its 10 Sefiroth and 22 interconnecting gates emanates from its roots (Ayn Sof) through four different dimensions, called "worlds." In the Kabbalah, these four worlds (from the top down) are Atziluth, B'riyah, Yetzirah, and Asiyah. They correlate with the spiritual, causal, astral, and physical planes of existence, although some may name or count them differently. Each dimension is a completely different vibrational level of existence. Following is a summary of the four worlds or dimensions of the Tree of Life:

- The top level, Atziluth, is the world where archetypes first form. In this dimension, the Sefiroth and letters exist in a premanifest form. It is a level of pure being. This level is the world of "emanation."

- The next world, B'riyah, is where the archetypes begin to differentiate. The letters begin to form words in this dimension. It is the level of the higher mind. This level is the world of "creation."

- The world Yetzirah follows with the beginning manifestation of the letters and archetypes of the preceding levels. This is the astral level of consciousness where the inner "psychic" senses of man/woman exist. It is the level of feelings. This world of "formation" is accessible to people in deep sleep and is visible in the dream state or meditation.

- The lowest world is Asiyah. This world of "making" is where the preceding worlds come together to manifest as physical reality. Duality is apparent at this level.

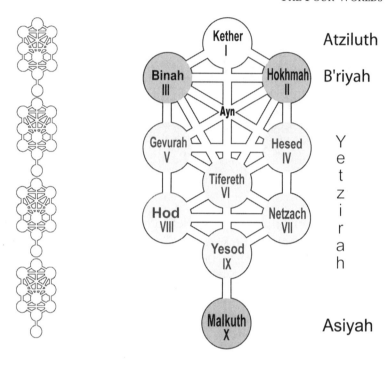

Figure 9.1 Vertical Trees   Figure 9.2 Four Worlds on the Tree of Life

The four worlds exist simultaneously and each contains a full set of Sefiroth and letter pathways. Each level is denser than the one above it, and the patterns in the higher realms reflect into the lower ones. Ultimately, everything manifests or expresses in Asiyah, the physical plane. Many of our problems actually stem from these deeper dimensions. Therefore, if we look at the body as only a physical reality, we ignore the three preceding dimensions and the many patterns that emerge from them.

Several schematic arrangements can be used to express the concept of the four worlds. In Figure 9.1, there are four complete Trees connected vertically. In Figure 9.2, the 10 Sefiroth are dispersed among the four levels. This shows us the nature of each world based on its position on the Tree. These worlds/dimensions are the subject of many Kabbalistic

100

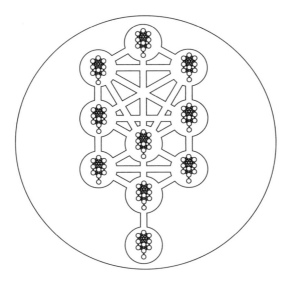

Figure 9.3 Trees Within Tree Within a Sefirah

texts and those interested in the philosophical aspect should seek out this information.

One characteristic of the Tree is that, as a universal hologram, it expresses in all levels of existence. Although there is only one Tree, it can be seen in multiple levels, so that there appears to be a full Tree inside of every Sefirah and a full Tree inside each Sefirah of the next Tree, and so on (Figure 9.3). This pattern is the same with the four worlds. Within each world, there are four subworlds and each of these subworlds can likewise be divided. This work began with a rudimentary knowledge of how to access the four worlds in the body. Over time, new expanded levels of the Tree have been revealed in much the same way as a tree puts a new ring of growth around its inner core each year.

The Number 4

Many things in human life relate to the number 4. There are the four corners of the earth, the four basic directions of the compass,

Humour	Blood	Yellow Bile	Phlegm	Black Bile
Element	Air	Fire	Water	Earth
Quality	Hot and moist	Hot and dry	Cold and moist	Cold and dry
Temperament	Sanguine	Choleric	Phlegmatic	Melancholic
Characteristics	Amorous, optimistic, generous	Short tempered, vengeful	Sluggish, pale, overweight, cowardly	Gluttonous, introspective, thin, sentimental

Table 9.1 The Four Humours

Letter	Y (י)	H (ה)	V (ו)	H (י)
World	Atziluth	B'riyah	Yetzirah	Asiyah
Location	Left Palm	Right palm	Right distal arch	Left distal arch
Shell	Spiritual	Causal	Astral	Physical
Nucleotide	Thymine/Uracil	Guanine	Adenine	Cytosine

Table 9.2 Correlations with the Divine Name

and the four directions of the medicine wheel. Early medicine studied the four humours of the body, which categorized physical and mental characteristics (Table 9.1). Rudolf Steiner talks about the four temperaments and the four dimensions of reality, which correlate exactly with the four worlds of the Kabbalah. There is much in science and human philosophy based on the number 4. The most sacred name of God in Judaism is the four-letter name, YHVH, יהוה. This four-letter Name is known as the Tetragrammaton. Some have translated this name as Jehovah or Yahweh. Each letter of the Name relates to one of the four worlds (Table 9.2). In the body, each letter relates to one of the four nucleic acid bases that make up the DNA.

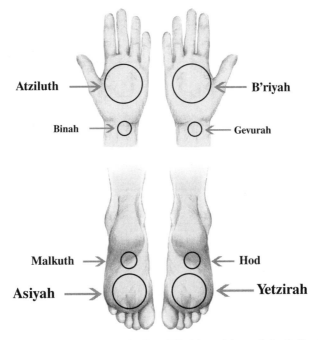

Figure 9.4 Indicators for the Four Worlds and four of the Sefiroth

Atziluth	Left Palm
B'riyah	Right Palm
Yetzirah	Right Distal Arch
Asiyah	Left Distal Arch

Table 9.3

The Four Doorways in the Body

The body is a miniature replica of a larger system, so it is possible to find analogs to the four worlds in the body. In fact, there are four doorways in the body that resonate to these worlds (Figure 9.5). Visualize the worlds as a four-story building with access to each floor through a special door. In addition, you need a key to unlock each door and these are the hand signs. The doorways are accessed by focusing on different areas of the body. Placing one's attention, concentration,

ATZILUTH	
B'RIYAH	
YETZIRAH	
A S I Y A H	Atziluth
	B'riyah
	Yetzirah
	Asiyah

Table 9.4 The Four Worlds with the Subworlds of the Physical Body (ASIYAH)

or visual focus on specific areas, tunes the body-mind to the worlds of the Tree. For instance, placing your attention on the top vertebra, the atlas, or at the base of your skull, activates the body analog of Atziluth. Raising your eyes 20 degrees to look at the point 1/2 to 1 inch above the eyebrows focuses you on B'riyah. Concentrating on the area of the heart activates Yetzirah in the body. The lowest world, Asiyah, is entered by focusing on the point 2 to 3 inches below your navel. Figure 9.5 shows the locations of these doorways. Note that the Tan Tien is

104

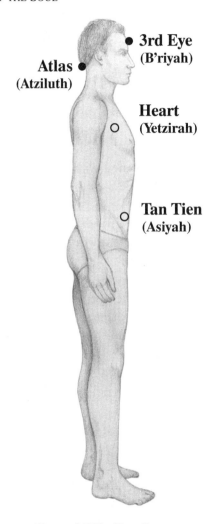

3rd Eye
(B'riyah)

Atlas
(Atziluth)

Heart
(Yetzirah)

Tan Tien
(Asiyah)

Figures 9.5 The Four Doorways

several inches into the abdomen, and the heart, of course, is in the chest. Chapters 13-16 detail how to use these principles to activate the worlds.

The Four Extremities

In Chapter 2, "As Above, So Below," we saw that there are 32 bones in each extremity, with each extremity correlating with one of

105

the worlds. Reinforcing this concept is the discovery that the points on the body that resonate to the four worlds are located on the palms and the soles of the feet (Figure 9.4). The points for Atziluth and B'riyah fill the center of the palms. On the soles of the feet, the points for Yetzirah and Asiyah are in the distal or front half of the arches. The points for the Sefiroth Hod and Malkuth are in the back part of the arches, near the heels.

In this work we are concerned with two levels of worlds. Table 9.4 shows the four worlds. Notice that the lowest world, ASIYAH, is subdivided into the same four worlds. This is the nesting quality of worlds within worlds. This book focuses on the physical world, or ASIYAH, and its complement of four worlds. This physical microcosm mirrors the larger system. In the pages that follow you will learn mudras to activate these four worlds of ASIYAH. As each of these worlds activates, touching its indicator on the palm or the distal arch of the foot will inhibit a strong indicator muscle. Table 9.3 reviews the indicators for the worlds. When the four worlds of ASIYAH become active within the body, then the doorway of ASIYAH, the Tan Tien, will test positive. In other words, a facilitated muscle will inhibit when one touches the area 2 inches or so below the navel.

The doorways are entry points to the four worlds. The palms and soles are indicators for the four subworlds of the lowest world, ASIYAH. Activation of the upper three doorways (Atlas, Third Eye, and Heart) along with deeper patterns in the Crown are currently being taught in my workshops. The purpose of this book, however, is to lay the ground work and this consists of bringing the physical body and its four worlds into alignment. This basic work is very effective and can balance many things. For many years this was my total procedure, so it is not necessary to have the deeper levels at this time. Nevertheless, those who develop an interest in this work will want to explore the next steps in workshops and future publications.

Experiments

With muscle testing, it is possible to verify the locations of the indicators of the worlds the palms and on the soles of the feet. Say the name of one of the four worlds and then challenge the latissimus dorsi or any other muscle while touching the corresponding point on the palm or sole. You can actually trace out the size of the points by moving your contact over the skin. Resonance between the word and the point on the palm or sole will result in inhibition of the muscle, causing it to appear weak.

In the same manner, you can test the doorways themselves. Say the name of the world and then test a strong muscle while touching the doorway. Having your partner focus on the doorway at the same time may be helpful in some cases. Again, inhibition of the muscle indicates resonance.

Katie

At a Sign Language of the Soul workshop, Katie told me that the reason she was taking the course was to find help for her chronic headaches and neck problems. She asked me if I could work on her in the class to give her special treatments for her condition. Instead, I told her that she would learn how to take care of her own health and I would guide her as necessary. As she learned and practiced the Tree of Life mudras in the class, she began to notice that her pains were going away. Each time we went through the mudra sequence she felt better. After the fourth or fifth circuit she exclaimed, 'how did it go away so fast?' She was accustomed to other people taking care of her and didn't believe that something she could do herself could give her that much relief so quickly. The stunned look on her face was priceless. The concept of putting her hands in different positions to relieve her pain seemed incredulous to her, yet she was experiencing it!

10
The 10 Sefiroth

The top Sefirah, Kether or Crown, represents the unmanifest potential of all existence and relates to Divine Will. Each successive Sefirah represents a different stage in the manifestation process until the 10th Sefirah, Malkuth or Kingdom, which represents the material plane of existence. They represent the stages that step down frequency from the most subtle level to the physical. The Sefiroth emanate as 10 sequential principles, and the use of circles to represent them is just a schematic for these great intangibles. The Sefiroth and their names are:

Sefiroth	English
Kether	Crown
Hokhmah	Wisdom
Binah	Understanding
Da'at	Knowledge
Hesed	Mercy
Gevurah	Power
Tifereth	Beauty
Netzach	Victory
Hod	Glory
Yesod	Foundation
Malkuth	Kingdom

Table 10.1 The 10 Sefiroth and Their English Names

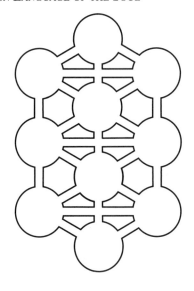

Figure 10.1 Tree of Perfection

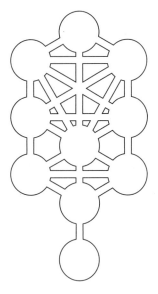

Figure 10.2 Fallen Tree

In addition to the 10 Sefiroth, there is a hidden, or invisible, sphere between Binah and Hesed at the level of the throat. This area represents Knowledge (Da'at) of the Ayn. Ayn means Not, which is the negative existence of the Source of Life. Da'at points to the original location of the Sefirah Malkuth, as it exists on the Tree of Perfection. Figure 10.1 shows the schematic representation of this Perfect Tree, and Figure 10.2 shows the commonly seen fallen Tree of Life. The Perfect Tree shows a symmetrical arrangement that indicates harmony, balance, and the perfected relationship of the 10 Sefiroth. In the fallen Tree, Knowledge of the Ayn is no longer located at the throat level, but it is now at the bottom of the Tree as Malkuth, since it has fallen from its original location. Knowledge of Oneness has fallen into materialism as long as we are under the illusion that we are separate from HaShem, our Source. When we experience this union, Malkuth disappears, only to reappear in its proper location at the throat.

The symbol of the fallen Tree we are using lends itself to a correlation with the body. Two forms of this Tree have been discussed

109

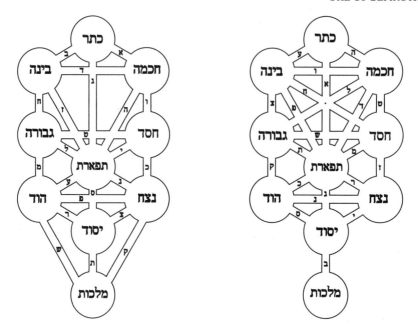

Figure 10.3 Two Different Arrangements of the Tree of Life

in Kabbalistic texts (Figure 10.3). The one on the left has pathways between Malkuth-Netzach and Malkuth-Hod. The Tree on the right has pathways between Hokhmah-Gevurah and Binah-Hesed. Notice also that the letter pathways differ on the two Trees. We will use the version of the Tree on the right (the Work of the Chariot version) because its pathways resonate in the body as demonstrated by muscle testing.

Figure 10.4 shows the Sefiroth superimposed on the human body. Here, the Sefiroth Hesed and Gevurah are at the shoulders and Netzach and Hod are at the hips. Some sources place Hesed and Gevurah at the elbows, and Netzach and Hod at the knees. In actuality, they test in both places, as long as the person you are testing focuses on one of the four doorways to the worlds.

This diagram shows the energetic locations of the Sefiroth in relation to the body, and it is possible to test them to validate this fact. Remember

110

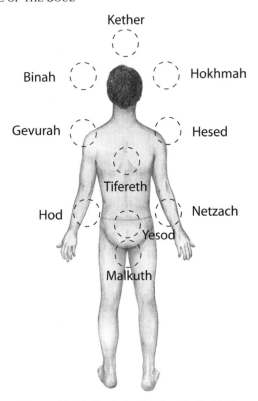

Figure 10.4 Sefiroth in Relation to the Body

that we are only looking at a schematic of the Sefiroth in relation to the body; they are not little circles on a piece of paper. The actual Sefiroth are infinite in size and represent universal principles, processes, and states of consciousness. At the same time, these universal principles are active within our own microcosm, and in this work, we are exploring the physical manifestation of such patterns within us. As a result, it is possible to test and validate their location in the human energy field.

Exercises

The Sefiroth have different names in each world, although the mudras are the same. Figure 10.4 gives the Asiyah names and energetic locations of the Sefiroth, therefore, your partner must focus on the

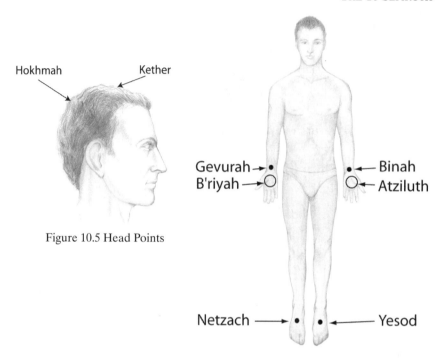

Figure 10.5 Head Points

Figure 10.6 Anterior Body Points

doorway to Asiyah, which resides at the Tan Tien, several inches below the navel. Find a person to test and then say the name of each Sefirah while placing a hand in the corresponding area approximately 5 inches from the body. The location for Da'at is behind the neck. Challenge the muscle, and if there is resonance (between the word and the location), the muscle will appear weak as long as your hand is in the area of the Sefirah. Touch the body at any of these points and there will be no resonance, because these are only the energetic locations.

Physical Location Points for the Sefiroth

We have just discussed the energetic locations of the Sefiroth. However, these locations are not of much use for activating the Sefiroth in the body. Each Sefirah has a hand sign, which activates it in the body

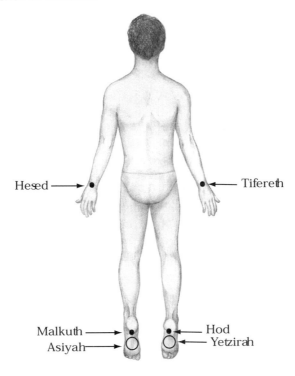

Figure 10.7 Posterior Body Points

when you focus on the doorway to one of the four worlds. The names of the Sefiroth also work, however, the names change in each world, so there would be 40 different names to remember. Eventually, 10 points on the body were discovered that resonate to the Sefiroth and, like the mudras, work in all four worlds. The points are shown in Figures 10.5, 10.6 and 10.7. They are located on the wrists, ankles, feet, and the top of the head (anterior and posterior fontanelles). Also included in these illustrations are the locations for the four worlds where they resonate on the palms and soles.

The best way to demonstrate these points is to start with a facilitated muscle and have your partner focus on his or her Tan Tien while you touch each of these points and say its Hebrew name. Then test the muscle, which should inhibit, indicating that there is resonance between the sound stimulation in the nervous system, the focus on the Tan Tien, and touching the area on the body. Holding a hand in the area near the body at these points will not demonstrate resonance. The points only work when actually touched. The physical location points of the Sefiroth are very helpful in treatment since you can just touch them instead of saying their names or employing the hand signs. They are very easy to use, and they produce dramatic results.

Summary

The Sefiroth have different names in each of the four worlds, so you cannot use the traditional names of the Sefiroth (Table 10.1) unless you are working in Asiyah. However, the hand signs and the physical location points for the Sefiroth work in all four worlds. Figure 10.8 shows the hand mudras for the 10 Sefiroth.

Notes on making the mudras:

❖ The flexed ring and little fingers do not touch the palm in the Kether mudra.

❖ There are two ways to make the mudra for Binah and Hesed. The thumbs may touch at the tips, or you can place the tip of one thumb on the other thumbnail.

❖ The mudras for Gevurah, Tifereth, Netzach, and Hod require that the thumbs cross at the proximal phalange (closest to the hand) or at the joint between the two bones of the thumb.

❖ It is important that the palms do not touch in the mudras for Netzach, Hod, Yesod, and Malkuth.

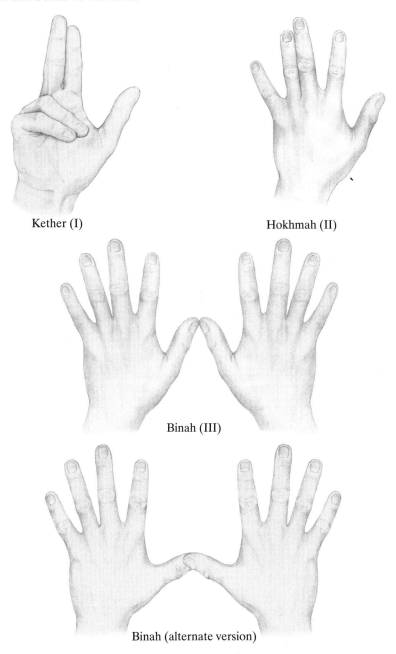

Kether (I)   Hokhmah (II)

Binah (III)

Binah (alternate version)

Figure 10.8 Hand Mudras for the 10 Sefiroth

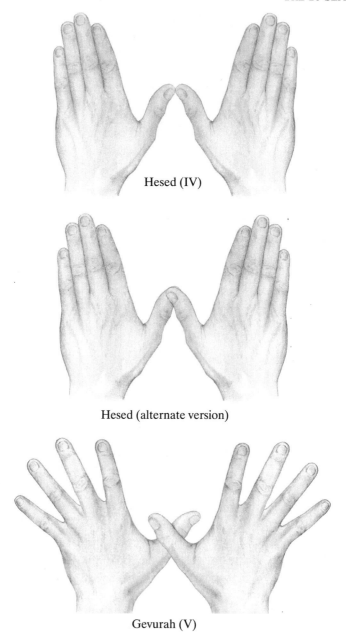

Hesed (IV)

Hesed (alternate version)

Gevurah (V)

Figure 10.8 Hand Mudras for the 10 Sefiroth (continued)

116

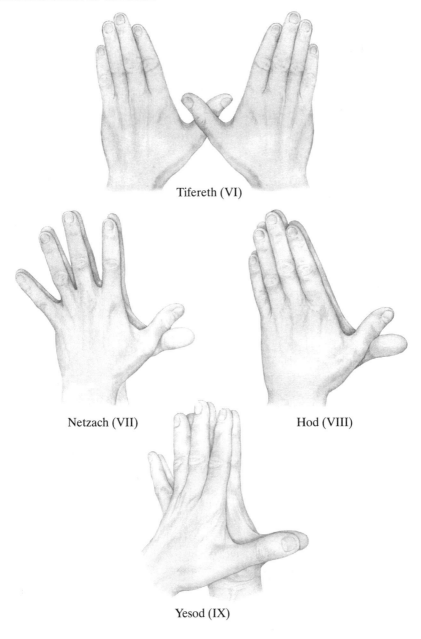

Tifereth (VI)

Netzach (VII)

Hod (VIII)

Yesod (IX)

Figure 10.8 Hand Mudras for the 10 Sefiroth (continued)

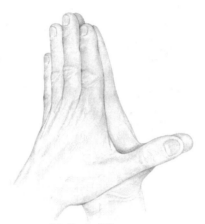

Malkuth (X)

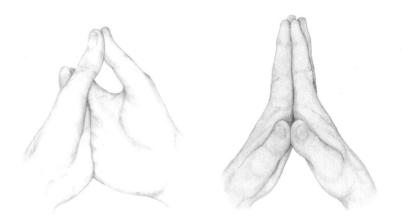

Bottom and side views of Netzach, Hod, Yesod and Malkuth
(The palms do <u>not</u> touch)

Figure 10.8 Hand Mudras for the 10 Sefiroth (continued)

118

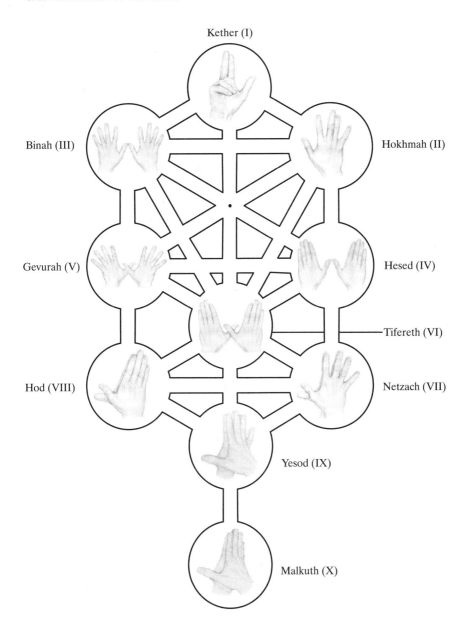

Figure 10.9 Hand Signs on the Tree of Life

"Twenty-two letters are the Foundation: three Mothers, seven Doubles, and twelve Simple. ...Twenty-two letters are the Foundation: He engraved them, He hewed them out, He combined them, and He set them at opposites, and He formed through them everything that is formed and everything that is destined to be formed." [40]

"In the beginning was the Word, and the Word was with God, and the Word was God." [41]

---

[40] Work of the Chariot Trust, *Sefer Yetzirah*, Chapter 2.1-2, www.workofthechariot.com.
[41] John 1.1.

11
The 22 Letters

The 10 Sefiroth are connected by 22 pathways or gates, which correlate with the 22 letters of the Hebrew alphabet. Therefore, each letter is a relationship of the two Sefiroth that they connect. The *Sefer Yetzirah* states that these 22 letters are the substance of creation. The Gospel of John starts with a similar idea, and it is these letters that form the Word. The *Sefer Yetzirah* correlates the letters with human experiences, the planets, the calendar, and directions of the compass. Everything relates to these 22 letters, since they are the building blocks of creation. The 26 letters of the English alphabet can describe all things. If there is a word for it, that word can be spelled from among these 26 letters. Likewise, the 22 Hebrew letters, as God's alphabet, embody all of creation.

In addition, the *Sefer Yetzirah* correlates each Hebrew letter with a different part of the body. The 22 letters break down into three categories. Three letters (Alef, Mem, and Shin) are the mothers of all the others and symbolically represent the first three elements of Creation. They correlate with the chest, abdomen, and head. Seven are called double letters (Beyt, Gimel, Daleth, Caph, Pey, Resh, and Tau) because each has two possible pronunciations. They correspond to the seven openings on the head. Twelve are called simple letters (Heh, Vav, Zayin, Chet, Tet, Yod, Lamed, Nun, Samek, Ayin, Tzadik, and Qoof) because they have only one pronunciation. They relate to the extremities and the organs. Table 11.1 shows the letters in these three categories, together with their various correspondences.

121

The Hebrew letters-body correspondences can be validated with manual muscle testing. The physical body relates to the lowest world, Asiyah, therefore, your partner must focus on his or her Tan Tien when you test these relationships. It is possible to touch an area of the body and then say the name of the corresponding letter to demonstrate a resonance. Those who are sensitive can feel it, or you can demonstrate it with muscle testing. Resonance results in the inhibition of a previously strong muscle. Test this with the 22 letters and their body relationships (Table 11.1).

Amino Acids

There are 20 amino acids and 2 stop signals coded in the DNA and these also correlate with the Hebrew letters. The correlation between the 22 Hebrew letters and the 20 amino acids plus the two stop codons of the genetic code is exact. I have found two researchers who have correlated the amino acids with the Hebrew letters, one of which tests accurate in the body.[42, 43] The correspondences that I have found to resonate in the body come from Steve Krakowski.[44] He observed a striking correlation between the Hebrew alphabet and the chemical properties of amino acids. One of the most basic chemical properties of a molecule is its capability to attract or repulse water molecules. Twelve amino acids are hydrophilic, meaning they are attracted to water molecules, whereas eight amino acids are hydrophobic, meaning they are not. One of these eight is methionine, which is also the start signal in DNA, so it counts as one of the three punctuation signals. This arrangement of the amino acids dovetails with the three categories of letters in the Hebrew alphabet: 3 mothers, 7 doubles, and 12 simples (see Table 11.1). In addition, the hydrophilic amino acids are polar in nature and the hydrophobic amino acids are non-polar. There are many other "coincidences."

---

[42] Hurtak, J.J. (1977). *The Book of Knowledge, The Keys of Enoch*. Los Gatos, CA; The Academy of Future Science.
[43] Krakowski, Steve, http://ddi.digital.net/~krakowss/index.html
[44] Ibid.

The amino acid-Hebrew letter correlations were validated by muscle testing for resonance between the name of the letter in Asiyah and holding the amino acid against the skin. Please do not take amino acids thinking you can activate specific letter pathways. This will not work and can be dangerous. It is better to activate pathways energetically.

Letter Pathways

The letters are the same in all four worlds, therefore, you can focus on any of the doorways to the four worlds when you test them. Focus on one of the doorways, say the name of a letter, place one of the two Sefiroth mudras that describe that letter, open the hands, and then place the other mudra. If this inhibits a strong muscle, it indicates that there was a resonance. You could also place the two sequential mudras and then say the name of the corresponding letter.

Hebrew	English	Mother Double Simple	Sefiroth (Asiyah)	Body Correspondence	Amino Acid
א	Alef	M	Kether–Tifereth	Chest/ribs	Stop
ב	Beyt	D	Yesod–Malkuth	Right eye	Valine
ג	Gimel	D	Tifereth–Yesod	Left eye	Isoleucine
ד	Daleth	D	Hokhmah–Tifereth	Right ear	Proline
ה	Heh	S	Kether–Hokhmah	Right foot	Tyrosine
ו	Vav	S	Hokhmah–Binah	Right kidney	Cysteine
ז	Zayin	S	Hesed–Netzach	Left foot	Serine
ח	Chet	S	Binah–Hesed	Right hand	Asparagine
ט	Tet	S	Hokhmah–Hesed	Left kidney	Threonine
י	Yod	S	Netzach–Yesod	Left hand	Aspartic acid
כ	Caph	D	Tifereth–Hod	Left ear	Phenylalanine
ל	Lamed	S	Hokhmah–Gevurah	Gall bladder	Arginine
מ	Mem	M	Hesed–Tifereth	Abdomen	Stop
נ	Nun	S	Netzach–Hod	Small intestine	Histidine
ס	Samek	S	Hod–Yesod	Stomach	Glutamic acid
ע	Ayin	S	Kether–Binah	Liver	Lysine
פ	Pey	D	Binah–Tifereth	Right nostril	Leucine
צ	Tzadik	S	Binah–Gevurah	Ileocecal valve + small intestine/ stomach	Glutamine
ק	Qoof	S	Gevurah–Hod	Spleen	Glycine
ר	Resh	D	Tifereth–Netzach	Left nostril	Tryptophan
ש	Shin	M	Hesed–Gevurah	Head	Methionine
ת	Tau	D	Gevurah–Tifereth	Mouth	Alanine

Table 11.1 Chart of the 22 Letter Pathways

124

Jim

Jim has been a patient of mine off and on for many years. I would repeatedly have to align his lower back and neck. It was always the same treatment. On one occasion, I decided to use the Sign Language of the Soul procedures with him to see if I could help him get to the root of his spinal instability. I gave him a spinal correction and found the appropriate nutritional supplements for him. Then I had him focus on his chronic back problem while he thought about his mother. There was no muscle response to this visualization. However, when I had him think about his father in relation to his back pain, there was an immediate weakening of all his muscles. Further discussion found that his father had died when Jim was a very young boy. I had Jim visualize a loving connection to his father while I applied the Tree of Life activation process. Not surprisingly, the low back showed up as needing correction, despite the fact that I had just given him an adjustment to this area. It took almost a dozen more corrections with various visualizations of the father who was missing in his life before no more pathways would open up. Not only did this treatment help his long-term spinal problem, but it helped him find some inner peace and security that had been missing in his life.

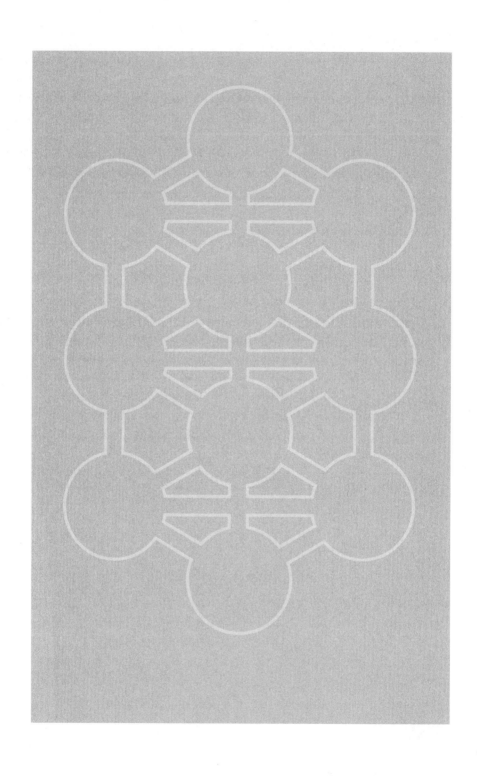

ACTIVATING THE TREE OF LIFE

The Soul

The Door of the Atlas

The Door of the Third Eye

The Door of the Heart

The Door of the Tan Tien

"And the Lord God formed man of the dust of the ground, and breathed into his nostrils the breath of life; and man became a living soul." [45]

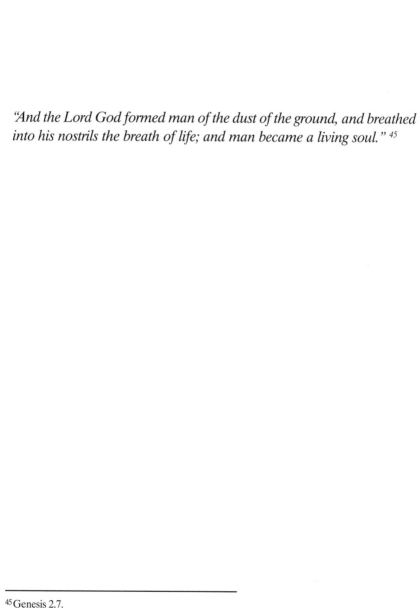

---

[45] Genesis 2.7.

12
The Soul

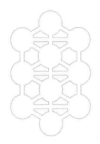

We now come to an exciting part of this work. So far, we have been developing theories and becoming acquainted with the tools. Now, you will start putting these concepts together to activate the Tree of Life in the human body-mind. You will learn a simple, highly effective method to center the nervous system to the spiritual blueprint, the Tree of Life. However, first we need a basic understanding of the Kabbalistic concept of soul.

Terms that relate to human consciousness may have various interpretations among different people. Only those who attain full realization of the highest levels of consciousness really understand the true meaning of the words that describe the indescribable. Those with full realization do not disagree with each other, even though the terms they use may differ according to cultural perspective or the purpose of the teaching. Therefore, when discussing the soul and spirit, it is necessary to be flexible in interpreting the written words and to know that direct experience of the higher awareness may alter one's perspective on these issues completely.

The term "soul" is not popular among scientists, who often use the word "field" instead. For instance, the ancients believed that magnets had a soul because of their magnetic ability to attract.[46]

---

[46] Sheldrake, Rupert (2001). Morphic Resonance and Family Constellations, *Systemic Solutions Bulletin*. London, England.

Science removes the word soul and replaces it with the word field. To scientists, it is the magnetic field, not the magnet's soul that attracts the iron filings. Likewise, we have gravitational fields, energetic fields, and so on. The soul/field is an attracting, organizing structure, even if it is unseen.

There is also a distinction to be made between soul and spirit. Spirit is the unseen force that moves through the structure of soul. The human spirit bears the same relationship to its physical body that God bears to His objective universe. The purpose of spirit is beyond our understanding. It is something we experience and witness, but cannot program or predetermine. Soul, on the other hand, is the structure that allows spirit to become manifest. In this work, we gently balance and align this subtle structure so that the spirit can more effectively express itself.

It should not be surprising that there is a different structure for the soul in each of the four worlds of the Tree of Life. The Kabbalah calls them shells or "husks," Qlifoth in Hebrew. These shells embody the spirit or consciousness of the soul at each level. Some systems refer to them as bodies: physical body, astral body, causal body, and spiritual body. These four shells emanate from the negatively existent roots of the Tree, which is the place of pure spirit.

In this work, we are facilitating the balance of the human body and energy system based upon the structure of the four shells. We do this in cooperation with the feedback of the person's body and energy system. The realm of spirit or pure consciousness is beyond any attempt to manipulate or affect. The higher Will, operating through the nervous system, always determines the outcome of what we do.

Following are the descriptions of the shells that embody consciousness at each level of the Tree.

• The deepest level of consciousness in the roots of the Tree is Singularity or Oneness, known in Hebrew as Yechidah. The statement "HaShem is One, but not in number" applies here. The roots of the Tree are completely different from any of the four worlds. They are negatively existent, which is a state that cannot be described or understood by the finite mind.

- The form of soul emanating from Atziluth, the top world, embodies consciousness as Neshamah. Neshamah means breath and relates to the "I am" consciousness.

  "And the Lord God formed man of the dust of the ground, and breathed into his nostrils the breath of life; and man became a living soul." [47]

- The soul emanating from the level of B'riyah is embodied as Ruach ha Qodesh, or the Holy Spirit. Ruach means wind, which is the movement of breath or soul.

- The next world down, Yetzirah, contains the astral body known in Hebrew as Geviyah. This is the world of feelings and this body provides our psychic senses.

- The physical shell of the soul is Nefesh. It resides in the lowest world, Asiyah. Nefesh means resting place, which is where the movement of breath or the soul rests for a time in a physical body. Nefesh relates to "chi" or the physical life force, and has to do with the instincts and actions of the body.

Activating the Levels of Soul

You are about to learn methods for tuning the body-mind to the multiple levels of soul using eye positions, breathing, mudras and/or words. The methods presented here serve to align the body to the higher frequencies, which is different from the deep attunement experienced in meditation. There are many ways for

---

[47] Genesis 2:7.

a person to attune himself or herself to the higher dimensions. Prayer, meditation, chanting divine names, visualization, and other heartfelt practices are the time-tested methods of spiritual attunement. Yoga, Qi Gong, and other systems also provide many ways to do this. However, the procedures developed over the next several chapters work as a very efficient, repeatable centering tool to align the body-mind to the higher frequencies. They are very useful when working in a healing session with yourself or others.

The higher soul is always living, open, and active, so we do not need to activate it. The purpose here is to tune the physical levels to the higher ones, and this is what is meant by the term activate. These methods will not necessarily open a person up to the soul in a way that will provide mystical experiences. Mystical experiences manifest according to a person's development and inner grace. These methods do not focus the entire consciousness on the spiritual realms; they merely serve to focus the nervous system of an individual on the higher dimensions, in a way that allows healing to occur. Merging one's consciousness with the Tree of Perfection can be a blissful experience, but that is not the purpose or outcome of these procedures. People often feel relaxed and peaceful from the Tree of Life activation, which in itself is evidence that the inner worlds have been touched.

This work depends on the concept that the body-mind contains structures analogous to the macrocosm. As a result, it is possible to align the body-mind to this universal pattern through resonance. The intensity of the attunement is individual, according to each person's level of development. The entire process is up to the person with whom you are working, or yourself, if you are self-balancing. Nothing is ever forced or manipulated. The mudras and words work with the energies of the person to create the effect. In fact, once you begin this process, there are no decisions to make.

Acknowledging One's Roots

Before activating the Tree of Life, it is important to acknowledge

132

the highest "dimension," the roots of the Tree, Ayn Sof. However, there is no physical or mental way to align to negative existence. It is only possible to touch the roots of the Tree through complete surrender to the divine in one's heart. Obviously, you cannot ask this of your clients, but you can do your best to maintain a loving attitude when working with them and they will automatically resonate to it. The more attuned you become, the more you can assist others in their healing. Therefore, begin the Tree of Life activation by maintaining a centered, compassionate, and loving attitude.

The Upper Worlds

The first part of the Tree of Life activation opens us to the higher worlds. This is a singular step and is the subject of this chapter. In the following four chapters, we will activate the four worlds of the body (ASIYAH), from Atziluth to Asiyah, or from the top to bottom.

The Eye

The following discussion lays the groundwork for the first step of the Tree of Life activation procedure. The retina of the eye can be divided into two general areas – the area centralis and the peripheral area. Toward the center of the retina is an area about 5 or 6 mm in diameter, called the area centralis, which consists of the fovea, a pinhead size area of very densely packed color sensitive cone cells, surrounded by the macula, which also contains primarily cone cells (Figure 12.1). The fovea, which makes up only about one thousandth of the retina, is responsible for hard-focused vision and much research has studied the tracking movements of the eye in relation to the fovea. The macula also provides good visual input although not as sharp as foveal vision. The rest of the retina is the peripheral area, consisting mostly of rod cells, which are less densely packed and are more responsive to light gradients and movement. Due to the predominance of rod cells, this area is the most active in night vision. If you place both fists out in front of you with arms extended, this should cover your foveal/macular vision and all the rest is the peripheral field.

Focused Vision

The world today thrives on focused vision. Computers, television, video games, and other electronic media all stimulate focused foveal vision. Few people are aware of the space around the television screen when they are watching an engaging show. Society teaches us to see and focus directly on our target of thought. It is a form of tunnel vision. When most people read, write, carry on a conversation, or deal with a task, they focus on the details and disregard what is going on around them. One downside to focused vision is that the ego is able to direct what it wants us to see as it can relegate unwanted information to the ignored periphery. This is why those with great intellects sometimes lack "street smarts." It is a different type of vision.

Focused vision stimulates the sympathetic nervous system and the pituitary glandular axes, which tend to stimulate the body and mind. This can sometimes cause tension to build up in the body, as people tire with prolonged visual concentration.

Peripheral Vision

Peripheral vision relies on the awareness at the edge of our focus. Peripheral vision is, therefore, less conscious, relying upon the night vision mechanism that makes us aware of subtle movements and shading. I once studied and then taught a method called PhotoReading.™[48] This course teaches a set of techniques called "whole mind reading" (not speed-reading). One part of this process involves diverging the eyes to diminish focused vision and allow the peripheral vision to take in the two-page spread of a book in one quick glance, thereby allowing a person to absorb printed information at rates limited only by how fast you can turn the pages. In other words, reading with your peripheral vision instead of focusing on the actual words, thus allowing a different part of the mind to take in the data. Other steps in the system help prepare the mind to receive the information, recall it, and so on. This technique of peripheral learning is surprisingly effective.

[48]Learning Strategies Corporation, 900 East Wayzata Blvd., Minneapolis, MN 55391.

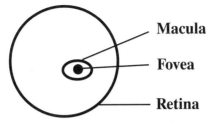

Figure 12.1 The Retina

Advertisers certainly know the value of stimulating peripheral visual pathways and they have made quite a science of it. They would not pay high prices for ad placement if the ads did not pay off. It is well known, too, that top performing athletes have excellent peripheral vision. In addition, you can observe that children naturally use their peripheral sight as easily as their focused vision. Anyone who has studied marshal arts knows that the key to most of the maneuvers is to maintain "soft eyes." By relaxing the eyes, which expands the visual field, it is possible to "see" the entire space with heightened alertness and readiness.

If you want to see a distant star, you need to look at the area next to it instead of directly at it. Similarly, people who see auras state that you must focus beyond and to the side of a person in order to see an aura.

Native Americans take nature walks using their peripheral vision. They focus on a point on the distant horizon and then begin to walk. Using their peripheral vision, they can avoid rocks, holes, plants, and other obstacles. This allows them to blend in with their environment, to notice the subtle movements of other animals, to hear, and to feel, the voice of the earth.

Years ago, I attended a NightWalking™ [49] seminar near Taos,

---

[49]Embudo Center, Explorations of the Dark, P.O. Box 181, Embudo, NM 87531.

New Mexico. In this workshop, we put on baseball caps that had a ten-inch rod attached to the bill of the cap. At the end of the rod was a phosphorescent bead that had a slight glow. We focused our attention on the bead and then began a several hour hike through the nighttime dessert on a moonless night. Focusing on the bead forced us to use our peripheral vision. The dark night became bright as we opened our peripheral (night) vision and it was easy to avoid obstacles and to negotiate often difficult terrain. It was incredible how it expanded the sense of self, and we all experienced many intuitive insights. I checked several of the other participants before and after NightWalking and observed that all structural distortions disappeared from their bodies (although they all returned the next day). I also observed the activation of their pineal glands.

This experience taught me that stimulating peripheral awareness activates the pineal gland, which has a balancing effect, even if temporary. Peripheral vision also stimulates the parasympathetic nervous system, which tends to calm the body and mind. This allows for more creativity and inspiration. Most of us stay anchored in focused vision during the day, and unless we meditate, take nature walks using peripheral vision, or engage in the creative arts, this part of our awareness is relegated to sleep.

In many ways the two types, focused vision and non-focused, peripheral vision, are opposite from each other. The first stimulates the sympathetic nervous system and the latter stimulates the parasympathetic system. The pituitary axes (pituitary-adrenal, pituitary-thyroid, pituitary-gonadal) keep the body functioning in activity and alertness. The pineal hormone, melatonin, has an inhibitory effect on these hormonal axes.

Pineal

The pineal is a cone shaped gland the size of a pea that sits in the middle of the brain. In addition to secreting the hormone melatonin, it also serves as part of the limbic system and thus connects to the autonomic nervous system. The limbic system is in charge of emotions, moods, feelings, and motivational behavior. Melatonin governs the diurnal cycle-the 24-hour cycle of light and darkness-thus directing our biorhythms. This occurs because light inhibits the production of melatonin, whereas darkness stimulates it. In addition, there is a direct neurological relationship between the pineal and light.

The pineal is often called the "third eye," and in some animal species it looks and acts like an eye and actually contains photoreceptive cells. Many people consider the pineal the doorway to higher consciousness. Descartes called it the "seat of the soul," and the ancient Greeks believed that the pineal connected them to the "realms of thought."

> *"The pineal gland is as a casement opening out into infinite seas and horizons of light, for it is the organ that in us receives the direct mahatic ray, the ray direct from the cosmic intellect or mahat. It is the organ of inspiration, of intuition, of vision."* [50]

When we go to sleep at night, the darkness activates the pineal and increases its secretion of melatonin. Melatonin has an inhibitory effect on the pituitary hormonal axes, thus allowing the body to rest and regenerate during sleep. As the psychic doorway of the pineal opens up, we travel into our dream world and beyond. In the morning, light inhibits the pineal, the pituitary axes reawaken, the body returns to activity, and we leave the dream world for waking consciousness.

Therefore, you can understand the importance of sleeping in a dark room (without nightlights). It should also come as no surprise that there are many health consequences for people who work nighttime shifts. Knowledge of this process is useful as we begin to tune the body to the higher realms, because it is necessary to find a way to access the door of the pineal, the door to the soul. The key to this is the discovery that concentrating on the peripheral visual fields stimulates the pineal gland.

---

[50] De Purucker, G. (1941). *Man in Evolution,* Pasadena, CA: Theosophical Press.

Beginning the Tree of Life Activation Process

The first step of the Tree of Life activation process is to withdraw your awareness from your body. There are numerous ways to do this, but the easiest way is to soften your gaze and expand your peripheral awareness. You can accomplish this in several ways, but the simplest is to focus straight ahead and then relax your eyes so that you can take in as much of the space around you as is possible. You could also place your hands out at the sides of your head and wiggle your fingers while looking straight ahead. You will see the fingers in your peripheral vision. Another way is to focus on a point at the end of a hallway, or room, and begin to walk toward this point. While you are walking, become aware of the walls as you pass them. Any of these methods will activate the peripheral fields, which opens up the door of the pineal to the higher worlds. This relaxes the mind, as it is difficult to think deeply about something if you have expanded your peripheral visual field. This process is one of opening, of letting go. It can also help you expand your peripheral view if you relax your mind. Soften your gaze, relax your mind, and then expand your peripheral vision some more.

If you want to work on a specific personal issue or a specific area of pain, you can use your mental/visual focus to concentrate on it prior to expanding your peripheral vision. When you open your peripheral vision, stop thinking about the issue or area of pain and allow your mind to relax. Inner resources become accessible through this process.

This simple act of expanding the peripheral vision tunes your body/ mind to deeper levels of the Tree of Life. There are more advanced ways to accomplish this activation, but they will be the subject of a future book. The advanced methods of activating the upper worlds of the Tree are also taught in workshops. For more information, see www. SignLanguageoftheSoul.com.

Summary of the activation of the upper worlds

❖ Focus on an area of pain, or a personal issue, and then let it go from your mind (this step is optional).

❖ Expand your peripheral visual field to take in as much of the space around you as possible.

13
The Door of the Atlas

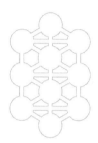

The top world is Atziluth (Table 13.1). The doorway to this world is at the atlas. This is the top vertebra of the spine. The base of the skull where it connects to the neck is also part of this doorway.

When you concentrate on a point six or more inches behind your neck, it activates the energy of the top vertebra of the spine, the atlas. If you then touch anywhere on this top vertebra, or the base of the skull, it will cause the inhibition in a muscle test. This special vertebra is ring shaped and supports the skull. Chiropractors have long known the importance of this amazing vertebra and many chiropractic techniques work exclusively with this area. It is no coincidence that this is the doorway to the top world of the Tree of Life.

The Mouth of God

The area behind the upper neck is the location for a special Sefirah. It is sometimes called Da'at, which means knowledge or realization. It is also called Reshith, which means first. This important energy area is considered a hidden Sefirah and is often represented by a circle with a dotted line. This is the hidden doorway to knowledge or realization of the Higher Reality. The great Hindu Master Paramahansa Yogananda called this area the "mouth of God,"[51] and he equated it to the medulla,

---

[51] Yogananda, Paramahansa (1946). *Autobiography of a Yogi*. Los Angeles: Self Realization Fellowship.

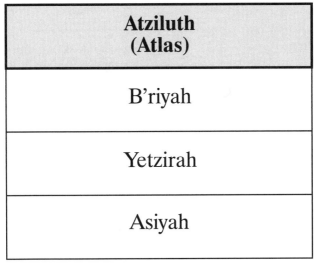

Atziluth (Atlas)
B'riyah
Yetzirah
Asiyah

Table 13.1 The Top World

which is the area where the brain transitions into the spinal cord. He claimed that the spiritual energy enters the body at this point.

Yod

The tenth letter of the Hebrew alphabet is the letter Yod (Yood). This letter is shaped like an apostrophe and is considered to be one of the most important letters in the alphabet. It's numerical value is 10, which is the quorum in the Jewish religion. It is also said that all other letters can be created out of the Yod. The mudra for Yod (Figure 13.1) is the precursor to at least six other mudras. This mudra is often seen in artistic renditions of the hands of saints and angels. This is the first mudra that you will use. Place it into your hands and then concentrate on the base of your skull or on the top of your neck at the atlas vertebra. Only a few seconds is necessary to initiate the movement of energy.

I Am That I Am

When Moses asked God what His Name was, the reply came, "I

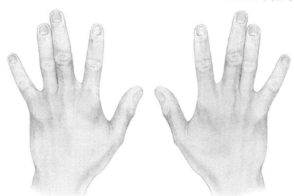

Figure 13.1 Yod Mudra

am that I am" or "I will be, That, I will be," Ehyeh Ahsher Ehyeh.[52] This Hebrew phrase is one of the most important mantras in the Kabbalah as it focuses one's being toward the roots of the Tree. Each Sefirah has a divine name or consciousness associated with it and Ehyeh is the name for Kether, the top Sefirah of the Tree. Some sources even state that Ehyeh represents the primordial point at the center of Ayn Sof out of which Kether and the other nine Sefiroth manifest.[53]

"When the concealed of the Concealed wished to reveal Himself He first made a single point: the Infinite was entirely unknown, and diffused no light before this luminous point violently broke through into vision." [54]

This single point is the manifest universe, including the subtle realms, and the name given to it is Ehyeh. The next step in the Tree of Life activation addresses this I Am point.

A very special mudra resonates to the words Ehyeh Ahsher Ehyeh. You build this mudra from the Yod mudra, which should still be in your hands from the previous step. On each hand, place the tips of the

[52] Exodus 3:14.
[53] Hall, Manly P. (1977). *An Encyclopedic Outline of Masonic, Hermetic, Qabbalistic and Rosicrucian Symbolical Philosophy*. Los Angeles, CA: The Philosophical Research Society.
[54] *Zohar*.

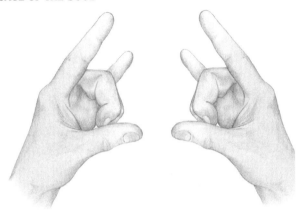

Figure 13.2 Ehyeh Ahsher Ehyeh or Om

middle and ring fingers to the middle joint on the thumb (Figure 13.2).
An interesting correlation is that this mudra also resonates to the word
Om or Aum, the Sanskrit word for the sound of creation. This is the
most powerful of all Hindu mantras and is often used in meditation.
The collective sound of creation is similar in concept to the primordial
point of creation. Therefore, this mudra resonates to analogous terms
in both Hebrew and Sanskrit.

Opening the Door of the Atlas

The activation of Atziluth is quite easy.

❖ Place the Yod mudra in the hands and concentrate on the area
at the base of the skull or the atlas.

❖ Then shift the Yod mudra into the Ehyeh Ahsher Ehyeh/Om
mudra.

This immediately tunes the body to Atziluth, therefore, touching
the left palm will cause the inhibition of a tested muscle.

143

14
The Door of the Third Eye

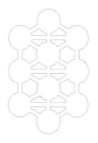

"If thine eye be single, thy body will be full of light." [55]

The next world we will activate is B'riyah (Table 14.1). The doorway to this world is the third eye. Humans have always looked upwards to the divine, whether in time of need or to express thanksgiving and devotion. The area of the third eye is important in all wisdom traditions. Observant male Jews place the Tefillin at the top front of the head and use it as a meditation and devotional focus. Hindus place a small red dot or bindhu just above the center of the eyebrows to indicate the singular eye. When people meditate, they usually focus their attention on this area. Raising the eyes 20° tends to relax the brain and induce the alpha rhythm state. Focusing on the third eye is more an internal concentration than a positioning of the eyes. However, focusing the eyes on this point creates the desired effect.

Breath

Breath is also important for unlocking the doorway of B'riyah. The movement and manipulation of the breath are at the core of most mystical systems, as breath is the prime mover of energy in the body. Tantric and Buddhist meditation, and Qi Gong, as well as all other protocols for meditating, employ special breathing patterns to

---

[55] Matthew 6:22.

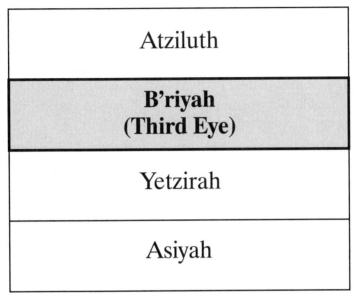

Table 14.1 B'riyah

center the body, calm the mind, and awaken consciousness. Breath work, called pranayama, can be useful if done in a way that honors the balance of the body. Anyone who studies voice or plays a wind instrument understands the importance of proper breathing. There is more happening when you breathe than just the exchange of gases.

Energy moves up the spine with inhalation and down the spine with exhalation. This parallels the fluctuation of the cerebrospinal fluid (CSF), which is found in the dural membranes (or dura), a set of membranes surrounding the spinal cord and brain. Within the inner portion of the dura is a fluid called cerebrospinal fluid. Produced in the choroid plexus of the brain, the CSF has a gentle circular motion within the brain and spinal cord. During respiration, the dura tightens at one end of the cranio-spinal system, and relaxes at the other end. Then this process reverses to create this rhythm. The effect is similar to gently tapping one end of a balloon full of water, which causes a small ripple effect that goes to the other end; gently tapping the other end creates the opposite movement. The CSF rhythm is between 6 and 12 cycles per minute. The respiratory cycle is 14 to 17 cycles per minute. The heart beats approximately 72 times per minute. Research into fluid dynamics reveals that after taking the rhythms of the heart, lungs, and the intrinsic movement of the fluid itself, into consideration, there is still a movement in the CSF that is unexplainable. Perhaps this is the life force itself. Many spiritual researchers have suggested that one's spiritual energies connect to the body through the CSF.

Cranial osteopathy, the craniosacral technique, and chiropractic cranial procedures (sacro-occipital technique and applied kinesiology) all work with the CSF and the dura to achieve balance in the body. The bones in the skull and the spine move with the breath. Everyone should experience these highly effective approaches at some point, but meanwhile remember that yoga postures, various breathing techniques, and even walking, positively affect the circulation of the spinal fluid.

Breath and Kabbalah

Breath is spirit. When we inhale, we inspire, or in-spirit. We literally bring the spirit in. When we exhale, we expire, or ex-spirit. We are letting the spirit out. In Hebrew, three words are used for spirit: Nefesh, Ruach, and Neshamah. Each is a different level of the soul (Chapter 12). Neshamah means breath and Ruach means wind, which is the movement of breath. Nefesh, which is the physical component of soul, means resting place. Breath (Neshamah) moves (Ruach) and lives in its resting place, or body (Nefesh). The Jewish concept of soul and spirit relates to breath.

The dualistic pattern of inhalation and exhalation enables us to live in the physical world. In other words, when we are breathing, we are in our dualistic state of consciousness. On the other hand, we move toward a singular state of consciousness when our breath stops at the transitions from inhalation to exhalation and from exhalation to inhalation. This may last only an instant in normal breathing, or a bit longer when consciously holding the breath. The effect is the same. It is a singular state, as opposed to the dual in-out movement of the breath.

146

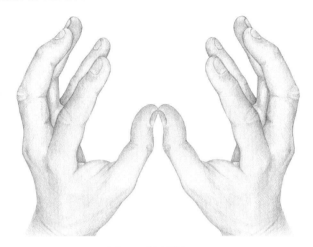

Figure 14.1 Yah

It moves the body away from physical consciousness toward the inner dimensions. The ultimate consciousness, nirvikalpa samadhi, is the blissful state of complete union that the yogi finds in deep mediation. It is a breathless state that the yogi can maintain for an indefinite period. The more slowly one breathes, the calmer his or her mind becomes. When the breath slows to a stop, a person's mind is in a heightened state of blissful awareness.

Yah

Since there are two active parts to breath, activating the third eye requires two mudras. The first mudra operates only on inhalation. First, focus on a central point 1/2 to 1 inch above the eyebrows (third eye) with your eyes closed. Then place the backs (not the tips) of the thumbnails together. The other fingers are open and apart from each other (Figure 14.1). There is no activation until you inhale. This mudra resonates to the word Yah or Yod Heh (YH) and correlates with an upward movement of energy in the spine. If you are working with a partner, he or she needs to do the focusing and breathing, while you make the mudra, or say Yah. Saying Yod Heh on inhalation accomplishes the same thing.

147

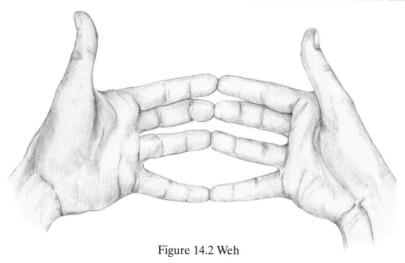

Figure 14.2 Weh

If you concentrate on the third eye with your eyes open when placing this mudra, it does not activate the doorway properly. Therefore, focusing on your third eye with your eyes closed is vital to activating the first half of B'riyah. The cerebrospinal fluid, the "river of life," tends to ripple upward on inhalation and this mudra, with the focus on the third eye, tunes the body to this upward flow.

Weh

The second mudra that activates B'riyah operates only on exhalation. Maintain your (or your partner's) focus on the third eye area, with your eyes closed, while you place the tips of your index fingers together and do the same for the middle, ring, and little fingertips. The fingers are separate from each other and the thumbs are open and apart from the fingers (Figure 14.2). Then exhale, as there is no activation until you do. This mudra resonates to the word Weh or Vav Heh (VH) and correlates with a downward movement of energy in the spine. Saying Vav Heh on exhalation accomplishes the same thing.

Again, it is essential that the eyes remain closed when placing this mudra and exhaling. The cerebrospinal fluid tends to ripple downward

148

on exhalation, and this mudra, with your attention on the third eye, tunes the body to this downward flow. This step follows the Yah mudra, so maintain the upward focus of your closed eyes, and shift the mudra from the thumb connection to the fingertip connections.

When you focus on the third eye, with your eyes closed, the Yah and Weh mudras activate the spinal system, the central core of the body, so you will find that they raise and lower energy here. Touch the right palm of your partner and test a strong latissimus dorsi muscle. If you activated B'riyah properly, there will be an inhibition of his or her muscle regardless of where he or she is focusing. Together, these mudras spell the name YahWeh or YHVH, the Divine Name.

Opening the Door of the Third Eye

❖ Close your eyes and place your attention on the third eye area, approximately $1/2$ to 1 inch above the center of your eyebrows.

❖ Place the Yah mudra (or say Yah) and inhale.

❖ Place the Weh mudra (or say Weh) and exhale.

Exercises

❖ Have your partner focus into his or her third eye with closed eyes and place the Yah mudra in your (or your partner's) hands. Then have your partner inhale and then resume normal breathing. Now run your hand up the body in various places and notice that the latissimus dorsi muscle does not inhibit unless you move your hand upward on the midline of the front or back. The third eye focus channels the energy into the central meridians of the body.

149

❖ Have your partner focus into his or her third eye with closed eyes and place the Weh mudra into your (or your partner's) hands. Then have your partner exhale and then resume normal breathing. Now run your hand down the body in various places and notice that the latissimus dorsi muscle does not inhibit unless you move your hand downward on the midline of the front or back of the body. Again, the third eye focus channels the energy into the central meridians of the body.

I taught the Sign Language of the Soul procedures to a friend of mine. Recently, her dog died, causing her much sadness, grief, and even some depression. I worked on her several times to alleviate her suffering and the procedures were quite helpful. However, it was not until she started using them on herself that she was able to completely resolve her emotions. She took a walk through the neighborhood where she used to walk with her dog and each time the sadness welled up in her, she activated the Tree of Life. By the time she got home, her whole frame of mind had changed. Instead of feeling the loss, she felt tremendous gratitude to her dog for showing her so much love. Remembering became a positive experience. Her entire attitude changed for the better, and she could then reengage life with a new outlook.

15
The Door of the Heart

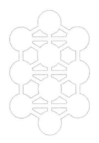

"Few are those who see with their own eyes and feel with their own hearts."

Albert Einstein (1879-1955)

The next world below B'riyah is Yetzirah (Table 15.1). The entrance to this world is through the heart. In this chapter, we will explore the energetic structure of the heart and its importance.

The Heart

On the physical level, the heart is a powerful radiator of energy.

"The heart's electromagnetic field is by far the most powerful produced by the body; it's approximately five thousand times greater in strength than the field produced by the brain, for example. The heart's field not only permeates every cell in the body but also radiates outside of us; it can be measured up to eight to ten feet away with sensitive detectors called magnetometers."[56]

It is no surprise, therefore, that the infant knows its own mother's heartbeat, which it has felt from the beginning of its development in

---

[56] Childre, Doc, & Martin, Howard (1999). *The Heartmath Solution.* San Francisco: HarperCollins.

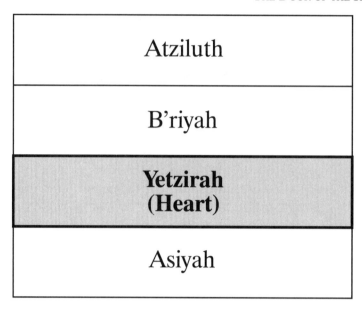

Table 15.1 Yetzirah

the womb. Even as adults, we retain this deep memory of our mother. Any human endeavor that activates the heart or comes from the heart has a greater chance of a positive outcome than one that does not. There is much research to validate this fact.[57]

Of all the organs in the human body, none has been the subject of as much attention as the heart. It is associated with love, compassion, and all things positive. Art, poetry, literature, and the stories that survive from generation to generation usually center on the heart. The goal in all wisdom traditions is to awaken the deeper levels of the heart. However, when love and compassion do not fill the heart, the dark desires of the heart create much pain and misery in the world. Unfortunately, there are many stories of this nature that also permeate our culture and others.

---

[57] Childre, Doc, & Martin, Howard (1999). *The Heartmath Solution.* San Francisco: HarperCollins.

We all have heard: "As a man thinks in his heart, so he is" or "As a woman thinks in her heart, so she is." It is not how we think in our heads, but what we think in our hearts that matters. The heart is the primary thinker and the intellect is secondary. However, this is certainly not how modern science and society view things. We worship the power and productivity of the intellect. Many of us think first, and if we feel at all, it is an after-effect. If the heart has 5,000 times more electromagnetic output than the brain, the intellect should be seen as a humble drive in comparison, and the truth of the matter, is that deeper forces operate within us at the level of the heart. These inner desires of the heart eventually manifest as the experiences and events in our life.

The Thymus

That wonderful feeling we experience in our chest when we are with someone we love is usually attributed to the heart. The feeling may actually stem from the heart chakra or energy center that resides over the chest, but the human heart gets the credit. However, another organ in the chest is also important. Just behind the sternum at the level of the second and third ribs is a small gland called the thymus. It is quite large in infants, but shrinks in size as the child develops. As this gland shrinks, its cells distribute throughout the body to set up the immune system. The thymus gland is one of the major components of the immune system. The importance of this gland is well known in holistic health circles and it has been shown that good emotional health, prayer, and positive visualization all tend to improve the functioning of this gland.[58] The function of the immune system is to distinguish between what is of self and what is not. Immunity, therefore, is identity. When you point to yourself, you touch the area of your thymus. For example, you would not point to your stomach and say, "It is my turn to sing." When something is determined not to be of the self, then there is an immune response. This is how the body recognizes an invading virus or bacteria.

---

[58] Dossey, Larry (1997). *Healing Words: The Power of Prayer and the Practice of Medicine.* New York: Harper.

Our deepest identity is a spiritual one. This is the point on which the immune system really pivots. When we are in contact with this deeper identity, we have incredible immune strength. This is why prayer tends to enhance immune function[59] and why people who have great love and compassion are able to work with severely ill patients without contracting the illness. Some great souls have worked with people who have leprosy, tuberculosis, or other highly contagious diseases and experienced no ill effect themselves.

On the other hand, we all have acquired and learned belief systems that operate within us, some of which are in conflict with our spiritual identity. Most of them are unconscious. When we have a poor self-image (identity) and other negative attitudes and beliefs, it affects our immune system. Much has been written about the physiology of stress and its effect on the immune system, so I will not repeat it here. However, the common task in all wisdom traditions is to clean and clear the negative self-identifications and to purify the heart. This makes sense spiritually, psychologically, and physiologically.

Although this chapter is about the spiritual heart, I have found that in the body, it resonates to both the heart and the thymus gland. This is also the location for the doorway of Yetzirah. If you have the capability to muscle test reflexes to both the heart and the thymus, you will find that they resonate together (not individually) to the heart chakra. Combining the electric power of the physical heart and the identification mechanism of the thymus gland provides the perfect way for spiritual consciousness to express itself.

I have observed over the years that many patients, in their inner hearts, have a deep, although hidden, agreement to their health problems. This is not to say that they want their illness or are the cause of it, but that the pattern for it to occur exists at a deep level

---

[59] Dossey, Larry (1997). *Prayer is Good Medicine: How to Reap the Healing Benefits of Prayer.* New York: Harper.

within them. It is unconscious. The work of Bert Hellinger is very helpful in understanding this concept. A former priest who became a psychotherapist, Hellinger has made some of the most important observations about the dynamics of the human condition that I have ever come across. He has mastered the understanding of personal and family conscience, along with the laws that govern how love flows in relationships. He exposes the unconscious dynamics within a person that predisposes him or her to have certain illnesses or life challenges. Hellinger shows how a person might unconsciously feel that he or she could benefit from having a serious illness. His work with family constellations and movements of the soul beautifully exposes the hidden entanglements that bind the heart.[60, 61] I highly recommend that you read his books, watch videos of his work, and become familiar with this important body of knowledge.[62]

Ahavah, Echad, Ananda

One mudra figures prominently in many books on the Kabbalah. This ancient mudra is still used by rabbis today (Figure 15.1). This mudra resonates to the Hebrew word Echad (the ch is pronounced as a hard kh sound), which means one. It also resonates to the word Ahavah, which means love. The numerologies of both of these words add up to 13, so in more than one way they are equivalent. To this day, rabbis place their hands in this position, over a person's head, and recite the traditional benediction.

> May the Lord YHVH bless thee and keep thee.
> May the Lord YHVH shine His Face upon thee
> and be gracious to thee.
> May the Lord YHVH lift up His Face upon thee
> and grant thee peace. Amen.

---

[60] Hellinger, Bert, Weber, Gunthard, & Beaumont, Hunter (1998). *Love's Hidden Symmetry.* Phoenix, AZ: Zeig, Tucker & Co.
[61] Hellinger, Bert (2001). *Love's Own Truths.* Phoenix, AZ: Zeig, Tucker & Co.
[62] www.hellinger.com.

Another word that resonates with this mudra is Ananda. This is the Sanskrit word for bliss. Therefore, we could say that the Hebrew word for love is related more to bliss than to other interpretations for the word love.

Moshiach

The Messiah, or Moshiach in Hebrew, is a major topic of Jewish scripture. Other wisdom traditions also speak of Messiahs who have, or will, come to the world to restore awareness of the Divine Plan. It is not, however, the purpose of this text to discuss the pros and cons of different teachers, avatars, or Messiahs. However, an interesting thing occurs when we separate the hands from each other while they are in the Ahavah mudra. It creates a new mudra that resonates to the word Moshiach. Starting with the hands apart in this mudra does not accomplish the same thing. Therefore, placing the Moshiach mudra requires two steps. First, place the mudras in each hand with the thumbs near each other, but not touching (Figure 15.1). Then slowly separate the thumbs until they are about 8 to 12 inches apart (Figure 15.2).

The act of separating the hands creates an opening in the inner heart, and, if you are sensitive, you should be able to feel the effect of this maneuver. The word Moshiach resonates to this mudra once you separate the hands. Prior to that, it resonates to Echad or Ahavah. Note that the mudra of the heart chakra is similar to Echad and Moshiach. The only difference is the crossed thumbs (Figure 15.3).

Opening the Door of the Heart

This step comes after the activation of B'riyah (Chapter 14). The following description is how you would activate Yetzirah within yourself. If you are working with someone else, he or she needs to do the focusing while you do the mudras or words.

❖ Focus your attention on your thymus/heart area at the upper chest, place the Echad/Ahavah mudra, and then slowly separate your hands 8 to 12 inches, keeping the mudras in the hands, to make the Moshiach mudra.

❖ Alternately, you could concentrate on your thymus/heart area and say the words Ahavah (or Ananda, or Echad) and then Moshiach.

Do this procedure on your partner. It should only require 10 seconds or less to activate this pathway. If you are in doubt as to whether you were successful, then touch his or her right distal arch and challenge a strong muscle. It should exhibit a state of inhibition. This indicates that Yetzirah has been awakened within the body. If you started with the beginning of the Tree of Life activation, touching either palm will also result in inhibition to a muscle test.

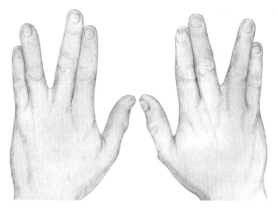

Figure 15.1 First Step of Moshiach Mudra (Echad or Ahavah)

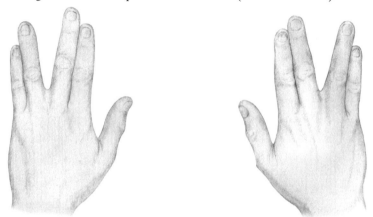

Figure 15.2 Second Step of Moshiach Mudra

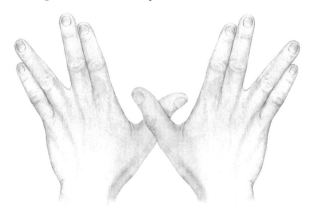

Figure 15.3 Anahata Mudra (Heart Chakra)

16

The Door of the Tan Tien

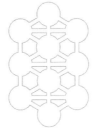

We now come to the last of the four doorways of the physical body, the Tan Tien. Once this step is done, the bottom world of the larger Tree of Life will be fully activated. In the next chapter you will learn how to balance the body and complete the 'circuit.'

Tan Tien

Eastern traditions such as Qi Gong, T'ai Chi, and acupuncture, all recognize one area as the center of the body, which is located 2 to 3 inches below the navel and several inches into the body (the location varies a bit with each person). This center is called the Tan Tien (Dahn Tee in), which means elixir field or field of vitality. Chinese medicine states that all healing comes through the Tan Tien, as it is the center of the chi or life force in the body. It has been called the "gateway of yin and yang" and "the root of Heaven and Earth." [63] This place is the source of movement in marshal arts and T'ai Chi and it is a focal point for meditation. The Tan Tien is the doorway to Asiyah in the body.

Shekhinah, Kundalini

The key that unlocks the doorway to Asiyah requires knowledge of

---

[63] Cohen, Kenneth S. (1997). *Qigong, The Art and Science of Chinese Energy Healing,* New York: Ballantine Books.

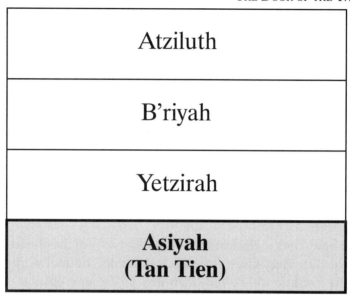

Table 16.1 Asiyah

Shekhinah. This is the Hebrew word for the feminine aspect of divinity. Many people mistakenly believe that the Kabbalah is a male-oriented system. Although it is true that only men counted for a quorum in Jewish observances and teaching (something that has changed in recent decades), the Kabbalah equally reflects the balance of both polarities. Shekhinah, the feminine principle, is the divine presence. Shekhinah, as divine presence, is, therefore, omnipresent. In many places, it is an alternative Name for God, since wherever God is, so is His Presence. The image of Shekhinah in the Kabbalah is of a queen, a bride, or a woman. Sometimes she is Sophia or Wisdom, which is another name for the second Sefirah, Hokhmah. In any case, Shekhinah is the Kabbalistic term for the Divine Mother.

The equivalent in Hindu Tantra is the word Kundalini. Kundalini is the spiritual energy that lies coiled at the base of the spine, like a snake, ready to awaken and rise up through the chakras. It is also a feminine force. The awakening of the dormant Kundalini is the goal of the yogic adept, through meditation, devotion, study, self-discipline, good deeds,

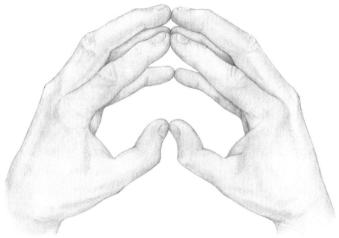

Figure 16.1 Shekhinah

and so on. A small amount of the Kundalini force is always present in the spinal system as long as life is present, but through these methods, the Kundalini force rises up the spinal column through the various energy centers and awakens consciousness at the different levels. When the Kundalini reaches the crown chakra, enlightenment occurs.

It is possible for the Kundalini force to awaken prematurely or out of balance with the individual's moral and physical development. Many things can stimulate the movement of the Kundalini force, and problems occur if it is more than a person can handle. A spinal injury, intense emotions, psychoactive drugs, and other chemical imbalances can all trigger premature release of the Kundalini energies. Excessive use of breathing techniques and sexual stimulation can also create problems in some people. If the Kundalini opens in excess of the person's ability to integrate the energy, it can cause psychosis. This is the reason why students of the inner life usually have a teacher or guru. The coiled snake at the base of the spine needs respect and careful handling.

Shekhinah is said to be exiled in the lower worlds of the Tree and seeks marriage or union with Her bridegroom in the higher worlds.

161

When testing the word Shekhinah or its mudra, it resonates to the area of the coccyx. This is not surprising since Shekhinah is the Hebrew term that is analogous to Kundalini. Therefore, it is important to awaken the Shekhinah/Kundalini in a way that is in harmony with the development of the individual. That is the purpose of this work. It is why we muscle test to see if a pathway is ready to open. Never force a pathway open. It is best to trust the wisdom of the body, and Wisdom is another name for Shekhinah. The methods taught in this book are safe because they work in cooperation with the nervous system and help to distribute the awakened energy safely. If a pathway is not ready to open, there will be no response to using the mudras/words. Everything is balance, and in this work, we trust the feedback from the body to keep us honest. If no pathways are present for balancing, then it is time to rest, eat, play, or do something else.

❖ To make the mudra for Shekhinah (Figure 16.1), place the backs of the tips of the thumbnails together and the four fingertips together. All five fingers are apart from each other and touch their opposites, except that the thumbs touch only on the nails, whereas the fingers touch on their tips.

If you experiment with this mudra apart from the Tree of Life activation sequence you can demonstrate that this mudra resonates to the area of the sleeping Kundalini. Touching the coccyx will inhibit a strong muscle after placing the Shekhinah/Kundalini mudra. The lower sacrum and coccyx is where the dormant Kundalini is said to reside.

Opening the Door of the Tan Tien

This step follows immediately after the activation of the Heart. Focus on the area 2 to 3 inches below your navel and several inches into the body. Then acknowledge the feminine spiritual energy with the hand sign of Shekhinah. This is the key that unlocks the door. Place the Shekhinah mudra while focusing on the Tan Tien. Instead of placing the mudra, you could say the word, Shekhinah or Kundalini. It generally takes only a few seconds to complete the activation of Asiyah, but it can take as much as 10 seconds.

Do the above procedure with your partner (he or she does the focusing, while you place the mudra or say the word for Shekhinah or Kundalini). Then observe the following indicators. Once Asiyah has been activated, you will find that touching your partner's left distal arch will cause inhibition in a tested muscle. In addition, you will also find that touching the Tan Tien itself will cause a strong muscle to inhibit. This indicates that the Door of the Tan Tien is now active in the larger Tree. In other words, all four subworlds of ASIYAH are now open in the body. It is not necessary to test the palm and soles after each mudra, but it is useful, especially at first, if you want to check to see if the activations occurred properly.

Summary of the Tree of Life Activation Process

The following is described as if you were activating the Tree within yourself. If you are working with someone else, he or she needs to do the focusing and breathing while you place the mudras. It can help the other person if you gently tap the area of the doorway when you ask him or her to focus on it. You can say the names of the mudras instead of placing them in your hands.

❖ Focus on an area of pain, or a personal issue, and then let it go from your mind. This step is optional and should be used after having activated the Tree of Life several times.

Initial Centering

❖ Expand your peripheral visual field to take in as much of the space around you as possible.

Atziluth (Atlas)

❖ Release your peripheral gaze to concentrate on the area at the base of the skull, the atlas. Place the Yod mudra in your hands, and then shift it into the Ehyeh Ahsher Ehyeh/Om mudra.

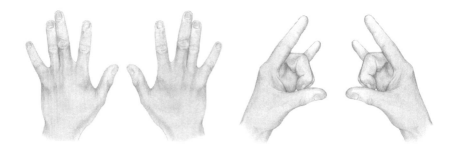

B'riyah (Third Eye)

❖ Close your eyes and concentrate on the third eye area, approximately $1/2$ to 1 inch above your eyebrows.

❖ Place the Yah mudra and inhale.

❖ Place the Weh mudra and exhale.

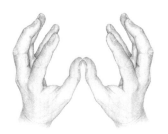 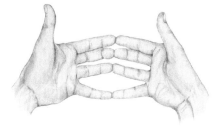

Yetzirah (Heart)

❖ Focus your attention on your heart, place the Echad/Ahavah mudra, and then separate your hands 8 to 12 inches, keeping the mudras in the hands, to make the Moshiach mudra.

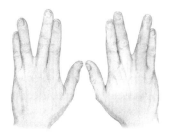 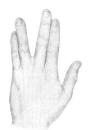 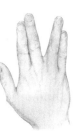

Asiyah (Tan Tien)

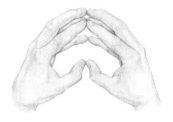

❖ Concentrate on the point 2 to 3 inches below the navel and 2 to 3 inches into the body (Tan Tien). Place the Shekhinah/Kundalini mudra.

17

Balance

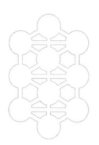

Tuning the body-mind to the Tree of Life is a profoundly centering experience. As a result, this centering usually exposes some imbalance that needs correcting. Be prepared for changes if you do this work! Left to its own, the body-mind flows along according to the direction in which it is heading. However, when a higher imprint is activated in the lower system, it causes the lower system to shift. This shift toward greater inner attunement allows some imbalance to surface. If we were totally in tune with the higher blueprint, there would be no need for this work or for healing of any kind. As this is not the case for most of us, we need strategies to help correct the imbalances that arise. This is where these procedures come into play.

If you have the ability to test the body or read the body's energy system in some way (chiropractic, kinesiology, acupuncture, etc.) then you should be able to find an imbalance that surfaces in the body following the Tree of Life activation. It is quite fine if you do not have this ability, so do not be concerned. If you began with a focus, then that is most likely what the body-mind is now displaying. In other words, if you touched your sore low back while doing the peripheral vision in the first step, then the low back would probably be the focus of the treatment. If you knew how to test the low back it would show positive in some way.

The balancing step completes the energy alignment that began

166

with peripheral vision followed by the seven mudras of the Tree of Life activation. Now you will find that one of the 10 Sefiroth will test positive. This means that touching the body point of one of the 10 Sefiroth will cause inhibition of a strong muscle. The other nine will demonstrate strength. If you prefer, you could test the 10 names of the Sefiroth, or place each of the 10 mudras to find the positive one. It does not matter which method you choose. Simply hold the active point until touching it no longer inhibits a muscle. You can also place the active mudra, or say the name of the active Sefirah This will initiate a movement of energy that will bring the body-mind back into balance. When the muscle returns to a state of strength you are done. Whatever surfaced from the Tree of Life activation will now be cleared.

I usually test a strong muscle after quietly saying the names of each of the 10 Sefiroth. The one that tests positive (inhibits the muscle) is the one whose mudra I then place in my hands. If you find that it is too difficult to figure out which Sefirah mudra is needed, then the easiest way to complete the sequence is to just look at the Tree of Life mudras (Figure 17.1). Have your partner look at the Sefiroth mudras while you monitor a muscle and when the muscle returns to a strong or facilitated state you are done. You can copy this picture so that you have one at home and at work. You can also purchase, for a few dollars, a 3"x 5" card that contains this image. See www.SignLanguageoftheSoul.com.

Following this balancing step you can start another sequence. Redo the Tree of Life activation process, as summarized at the end of Chapter 16. Then treat with one of the Tree of Life Mudras, points, or use the image of the mudras on the Tree. Continue activating the Tree and balancing the system until no more pathways will open. You can tell that the body has had enough when activating the door of the atlas does not cause an inhibition of a muscle when touching the left palm. Each step in the Tree of Life activation process causes a brief inhibition in a strong muscle as the body shifts to the new perspective associated with the mudra. If you have a free hand for testing, or are quick enough, you can verify it this way as well.

Working with Children

The Tree of Life activation described here is quite safe for using with children. Tap the points to help them focus and make a game out of it. I will sometimes do the breathing for young children. The Tree of Life mudra image is quite balancing for children and just looking at this illustration is healing to them. It can be helpful to place a poster of this image on the wall of your child's room.

Robert

Robert hurt his left knee while lifting heavy boxes and had been limping for several months. He could not fully lock his knee straight. Evaluation of the knee did not reveal any swelling or obvious ligament damage, although damage could not be totally ruled out. Using the Sign Language of the Soul balancing procedures, I stabilized his pelvic imbalance and several muscles around the knee. Upon standing, he still was unable to straighten his leg fully. I tested all the muscles around his left knee and found one small muscle that was still dysfunctional and then focused a balancing procedure on this specific area. After this correction, he was able to lock his knee straight without any problem.

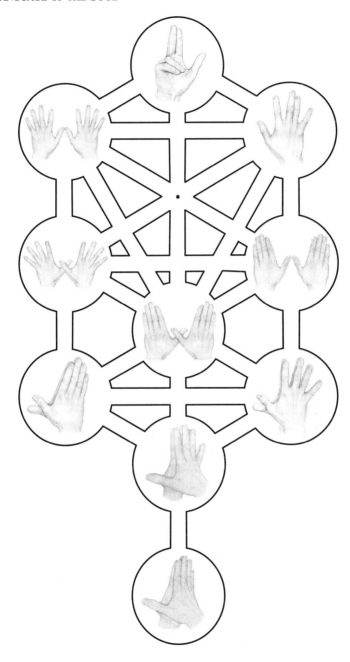

Figure 17.1 Hand Signs on the Tree of Life

169

18
Going Deeper

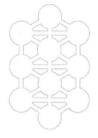

Some books on the Kabbalah devote an entire chapter to each pathway of the Tree of Life. This book, however, focuses on a healing application of this inner knowledge. I have tried to give just enough information to allow you to follow the concepts behind the various mudras/words and eventually use them as healing tools. You now have a way to activate the Tree of Life. Just applying these methods will provide most people with a new level of balance and integration. But healing is more than a series of techniques. It requires a deep respect for and understanding of the issues that keep humankind entrapped in limited thinking and experience. Therefore, we must search for ways to use these methods to clear deeper patterns that do not readily surface in the system. Some traumas that we have experienced do not readily reveal themselves for treatment. This chapter discusses how to expose these hidden wounds so that they might receive healing.

Adaptation

The human body and mind are wonderful adapters, for better or worse. We can adapt to almost anything. Our ability to adapt allows us to continue with life even in devastating circumstances. On the other hand, we sacrifice a part of us when we have to adapt to a difficult situation; it is like throwing one person overboard to keep the whole boat afloat. Moreover, in order to survive, we often forget that we had to adapt to something. This is the ultimate "successful" adaptation. When it comes time to heal and reunite the parts of us that have been "thrown overboard," it can be difficult to get past the coping mechanism of forgetting. For example, as adults, we may not consciously remember the harmful messages of childhood. However, a deeper part of us always does, and these unresolved issues silently direct our actions in ways that are usually contrary to our better judgment.

Often the traumas we experience are irreversible, as in cases of death and other losses. Nevertheless, it is possible to reconcile loss through deeply honoring, and agreeing with, fate's plan for us. There is no other healthy choice. Anything less leads to adaptation as a way of life, even when circumstances no longer require it, even when it is actually detrimental. Forgetting can be a good short-term stabilizing factor, but only remembering and being fully conscious with an open heart can lead us to freedom.

Although we cannot change the past, the imprint of a trauma and its ongoing effect can be released from the body-mind. Patterns of all of our adaptations exist within us, and it is just a matter of finding a safe way to bring them to the surface. This programmed information is located in the various pathways on the Tree of Life as blocks, toxicity, and confusion. In the physical body, they exist as the many imbalances that cause us discomfort and illness. In life, they show up in the dysfunctions of our relationships and experiences.

It has been my experience that it is really quite easy to balance the body. The balancing method taught in this book will correct most structural or energetic distortions, quickly and effectively. The more difficult task is exposing the areas that need balancing and getting past the defenses and adaptations of the body-mind. This is where the healer needs to become the detective in order to get to the core of the issue. It helps to have good powers of observation and intuition. Most of all, however, it requires that the healer face and resolve his or her own traumas and other life issues. This gives a person the objectivity to see and feel the needs of others.

171

It is necessary to bring healing to areas of pain and trauma. Those areas that are already in tune with the higher patterns do not need help. Although this sounds obvious, it is the key to deeper healing. It is important to meditate, pray, and develop a rich, positive inner life. However, it is equally important not to wall off our shadow side. It is nice to feel good, loving, and in tune when we are in meditation, but it does not serve us well if we return to the world to cheat, ignore suffering, and create other mischief. Therefore, we must learn to embrace our shadow self from the perspective of our loving soul, place the negative experience on the Tree of Life, and then balance it.

In cases of trauma, the body quickly defends itself with a barrage of hormones that ensure short-term survival, but ignore long-term consequences. This is adaptation. The hormones mask the illness or trauma so that it is not visible. Therefore, when you are working on someone who has experienced a trauma, physical or emotional, it is often necessary to have the person visualize the trauma, touch the area(s) involved, assume the appropriate posture, and hear, see, feel, and smell anything related to the incident. As soon as the mind revisits the injury, the body says, "I remember this," and it begins to exhibit the internal response that occurred at the time. Now that the body shows the response to the injury, activate the Tree of Life and then look at the image of the mudras on the Tree. Several sequences of centering and balancing may be necessary, with different variations of the visualization, to release the trauma from the body-mind. It is helpful to test the strong latissimus dorsi muscle, and then have the person visualize the insult, accident or injury and retest the muscle. If the muscle inhibits, do the Tree of Life activation and then activate the positive Sefirah or look at the image of the mudras on the Tree

Have your client (do this on yourself as well) visualize any traumas experienced as a child. Visualize the tragedy surrounding the World Trade Center, and feel the fears that we all have for our security. Have your client focus on his or her spiritual ideal while at the same time recalling a painful event. Bring these disparate images together to expose the incongruence in the system. After each of these images, do

172

the Tree of Life activation, and then look at the Sefiroth mudras on the Tree. In this way, you can extend the reach of these healing procedures to areas that might not volunteer for treatment. It is a way to shine the inner light on the shadow side of our consciousness. The methods taught in this book are powerful balancing tools, and it is up to you to learn how to apply them in a way that will maximize the outcome you want to achieve. You will be pleasantly surprised by the effectiveness of this method.

One way to work with yourself using these techniques is to focus on your dreams soon after you awaken in the morning. The Talmud says that a "dream that is not understood is like a letter unopened." This is an excellent technique for integrating the unconscious patterns of the mind. Focus on the images and feelings of the dream, do the Tree of Life activation, and look at the Tree of Life mudras, or place the active mudra in your hands.

It is also useful to spend a few minutes reviewing your day just before bedtime. Any stressful images from the day can be your focus. Center yourself to the Tree of Life after visualizing the stress, fear, guilt, or anger of the day. Then use the Tree of Life mudra image to balance yourself. This can be a good prelude to meditation as it can help calm and clear the mind. Meditation is time spent in quiet inner communion, not for working out problems. Save your problems for a contemplation period after meditation.

You can use these procedures for almost any imbalance that will cause a strong muscle to inhibit. For instance, if you have an allergy, it is possible to taste or smell the offending agent (if you are highly sensitive, you can just place the substance against your skin) and then do the Tree of Life activation followed by one of the mudras. It may take a number of these centering and balancing procedures before you resolve the reactivity of the body and nutritional, dietary, and detoxification protocols may also be necessary.

Many of our deepest problems stem from our family relationships.

173

Often, the traumas of our ancestors have a dramatic impact on our lives. Understanding family loyalty (love) is paramount to true healing. I touched briefly on the work of Bert Hellinger in Chapter 15, but I will reiterate here how important it is to understand the "Orders of Love" and other dynamics of family systems.[64] Deep unconscious forces that operate on us originate in the collective soul of our family. When you combine an understanding of these patterns with the balancing methods taught here, the sky is the limit to what you can achieve.

In addition to focusing on problem areas, it is highly recommended that you also spend time placing your full attention upon your spiritual ideal. Seek inwardly for a greater personal connection to this ideal and then see if the Tree of Life activation is possible. Make positive spiritual statements, such as "All my experiences are a direct gift from God to my soul," or "I claim the patience of my soul," and then see if the Tree of Life patterns can be activated. Say these statements while focusing on an area of stress in your life. Be creative in finding new patterns to support your areas of weakness. These methods can be useful in helping you to establish new habit patterns in your thinking and feeling life.

I suggest that you use these procedures daily for a month and observe the positive changes in your life. You may only need to do a few circuits each day, but if you are creative in searching your memory for the past traumas and for your weaknesses, you might be quite busy.

You will also probably find that there is a limit to what you can accomplish with the Sign Language of the Soul procedures. At some point most people require some form of nutritional support, whether it is more water, detoxification, or specific vitamin or mineral supplementation. You will have to seek assistance in this area. The same goes for physical adjustment of the spine, massage, or acupuncture. Tailor a program that fits your individual needs.

If you plan to use these methods with others as a healer or therapist, it

---

[64] Hellinger, Bert (2002). *Insights.* Heidelberg, Germany: Carl-Auer-Systeme Publishers.

is essential that you apply them to yourself first. "Healer, heal thyself" is the adage. If applied properly, these procedures have great potential to balance and heal. It is important that those who use them maintain a humble, compassionate attitude toward service to others. These procedures give us great scope in healing since we can navigate the Tree of Life, but we must always keep in mind that the roots are what keep the Tree alive. This is where healing comes from, and all credit for that healing goes to HaShem.

Sarah

Sarah, a 71-year-old woman, had severe osteoporosis resulting in spine and joint deformity. Since she had many fractures in her spine, I was not going to be performing any strong physical adjustments. The Sign Language of the Soul procedures were an excellent resource for her. They provided a gentle method to balance her system. I was able to keep her relatively pain free, with regular visits, doing nothing more than the Tree of Life activation and the Tree of Life mudras.

19

Final Thoughts

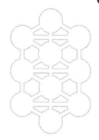

Our culture is enamored of technology and most of us are heavily reliant on it, whether we are wedded to our computers, cell phones, palm pilots, or all of the above. Medicine is no different and, in fact, probably leads the charge toward using the newest technologies. The MRI scans the body; the PET scan gives us amazing pictures of the brain; SQUID magnetometers scan the biomagnetic fields that emanate from us; instruments that measure heart rate variability show us our emotional health risks, and so on. Sophisticated electronic instruments can evaluate the status of the acupuncture meridians and send customized therapeutic treatment back to the body. What these wonderful technologies have in common is that they read and measure the energy fields of the body, using radio waves, magnetism, biomagetism, positrons, and electrons. Some of these machines rely upon quantum physics in their design. Here is the interface of technology and energy medicine and these machines are providing "mainstream" support for the efficacy, if not the theories, of many holistic therapies.

One drawback of technology is that it is expensive and not available to everyone; another, is that it often comes between the physician and patient. Doctors may spend more time obtaining and evaluating the technological results than actually being with the patient. In addition, managed care and its treatment guidelines have created a situation in which few physicians can take the time to investigate alternatives or to be creative in finding more than a palliative solution to a person's health problem. No wonder so many people have gravitated toward complementary health providers. People are learning that they have to take responsibility for their own health, doing research in books and on the Internet and pursuing options such as yoga, T'ai Chi, Qi Gong, meditation, exercise, and nutritional therapies. It is clear that bodywork (chiropractic, massage, Rolfing, and Feldenkrais) and energetic therapies (homeopathy and acupuncture) can help people function better in a complicated, stressful world.

What you have been learning in this book is a new way to balance the body, a soft technology that relies on the hands and the heart. There is a hierarchy in the nervous system, just as there is one in the universe. When we look at a problem from the highest vantage point, we get the best perspective on how to move toward a solution. By tuning the body to this higher view, our therapeutic success rate improves. A person only has to work with this system for a short while in order to gain great confidence in the ability of the body to heal and resolve very complex health and emotional issues.

We have explored many things that correlate with the Tree of Life pattern, and have seen how they can be applied to the body in a therapeutic manner. These correlations serve to remind us that everything is an expression of an unseen reality that is neither random nor arbitrary. Although we may not understand the reasons behind all of our experiences in life, we may be certain that the structure within which we live is organized, multidimensional, intelligent, and purposeful. And when we align ourselves with this internal structure of the soul, our spirit has a greater chance to express itself in a harmonious manner. When integrated into the body-mind, the patterns of our deeper soul are always soothing and healing.

There are many wonderful holistic healing methodologies, but none addresses the body-mind-soul in the way that this system does. You may still need nutritional therapy, homeopathy, chiropractic, acupuncture, or a host of other beneficial therapies, but none of these other approaches have the same impact as the Sign Language of the Soul procedures.

You now have tools to research your own Tree of Life. But, you must do the work. I encourage you to find a partner with whom you can practice. Have fun and experiment, but always return to the Tree of Life activation process and the Sefiroth mudras. These patterns have been well tested. If what you want to accomplish is greater balance in your body or some other aspect of your life, then these procedures should be quite useful to you. These methods can also help you with your spiritual attunement. However, the Tree of Life patterns presented in this book are just the beginning of the journey. They represent the connections to the body-mind. There are many deeper levels within the being, which are beyond what has been presented here. If you wish to investigate these deeper levels within yourself, you must travel the spiritual path and the safest method of inner development is always through deep meditation and devotional practices. However, be forewarned that there are certain dangers without a proper guide, so seek support from qualified teachers. (Hint: a qualified teacher supports your growth and does not require allegiance to his or her belief system, popularity, or pocketbook.)

The sequencing of the mudras has been constantly evolving over the last 20 years, although the patterns presented here have been consistently stable and effective. Even so, this is not the end of the road. New insights continue to move the work forward as deeper levels of the Tree reveal themselves. There is even more to learn about how to creatively apply these procedures than there is in learning them and that will be the subject of a future book. For those who are interested in future evolutions in this work, go to my Website www.SignLanguageoftheSoul.com. I will also offer ongoing workshops on this subject, which will include the advances in the work.

E-mail me your questions and experiences with this work at DrDale@SignLanguageoftheSoul.com.

I wish you great success as you balance yourself to your inner Tree of Life.

Appendix I
Hand Signs

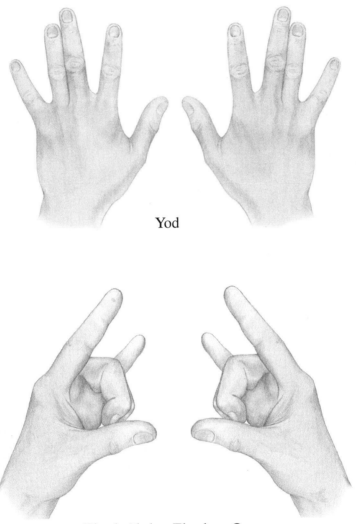

Yod

Ehyeh Ahsher Ehyeh or Om

179

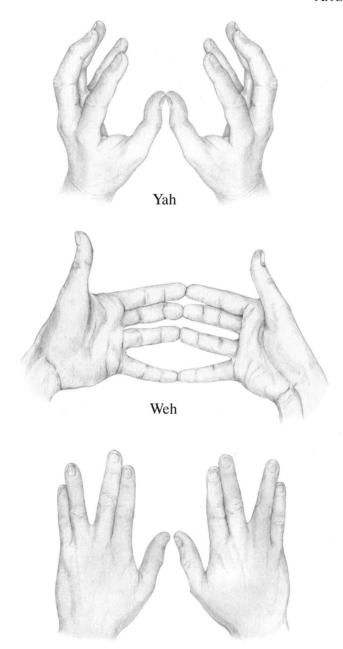

Yah

Weh

Echad or Ahavah

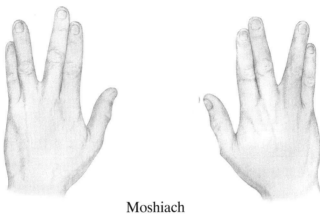

Moshiach

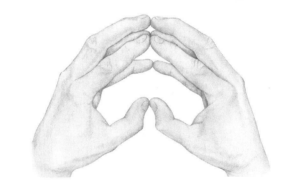

Shekhinah or Kundalini

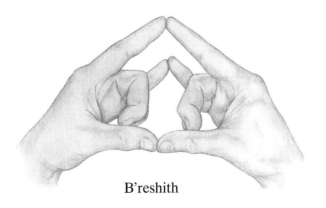

B'reshith

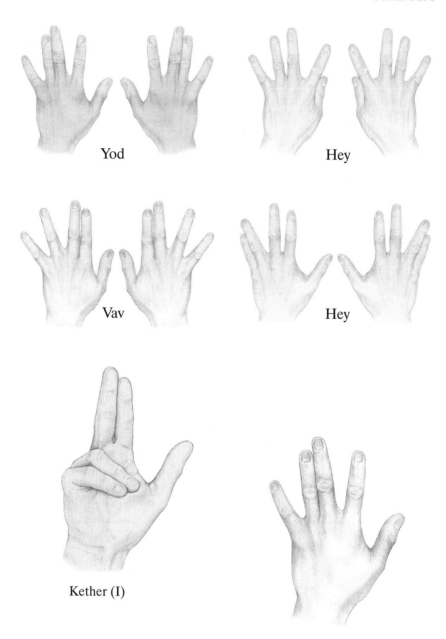

Yod

Hey

Vav

Hey

Kether (I)

Hokhmah (II)

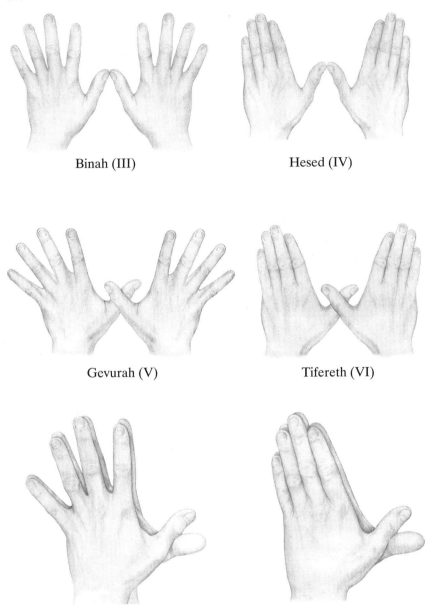

Binah (III)

Hesed (IV)

Gevurah (V)

Tifereth (VI)

Netzach (VII)

Hod (VIII)

Above: Side view of Netzach and Hod

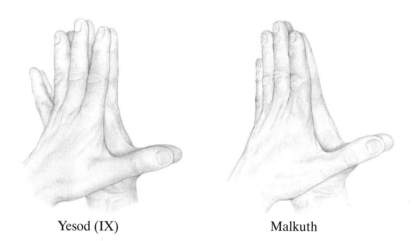

Yesod (IX)　　　　　　Malkuth

Above: Side view of Yesod, Malkuth

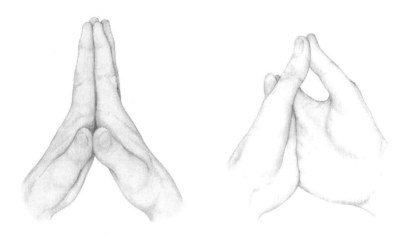

Above: Side and bottom view of Netzach, Hod, Yesod, Malkuth

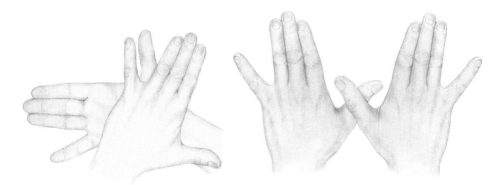

Equivalent mudras for Ajna Chakra

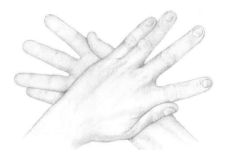

Visuddha Chakra

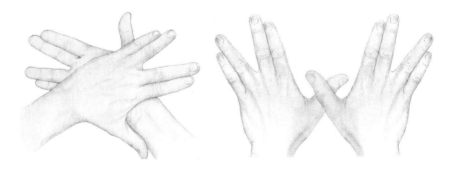

Equivalent Mudras for the Anahata Chakra

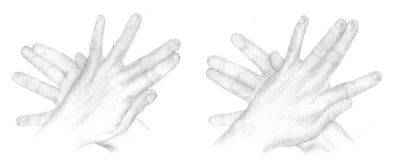

Manipura Chakra   Svadisthana Chakra

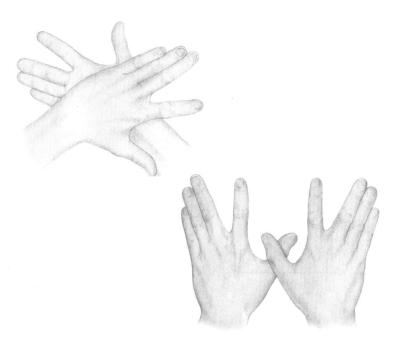

Equivalent Mudras for the Muladhara Chakra

Summary of the
Tree of Life Activation Process

The following is described as if you were activating the Tree within yourself. If you are working with someone else, he or she needs to do the focusing and breathing while you place the mudras. It can help the other person if you gently tap the area of the doorway when you ask him or her to focus on it. You can say the names of the mudras instead of placing them in your hands.

❖ Focus on an area of pain, or a personal issue, and then let it go from your mind. This step is optional and should be used after having activated the Tree of Life several times.

Initial Centering

❖ Expand your peripheral visual field to take in as much of the space around you as possible.

Atziluth (Atlas)

❖ Release your peripheral gaze to concentrate on the area at the base of the skull, the atlas. Place the Yod mudra in your hands, and then shift it into the Ehyeh Ahsher Ehyeh/Om mudra.

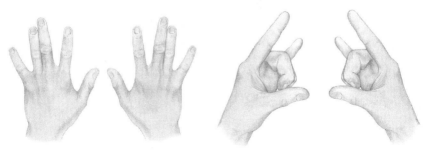

B'riyah (Third Eye)

❖ Close your eyes and concentrate on the third eye area, approximately 1/2 to 1 inch above your eyebrows.

❖ Place the Yah mudra and inhale.

❖ Place the Weh mudra and exhale.

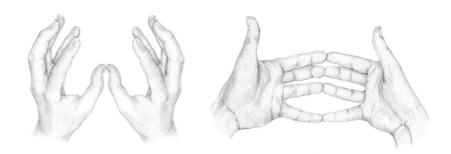

Yetzirah (Heart)

❖ Focus your attention on your heart, place the Echad/Ahavah mudra, and then separate your hands 8 to 12 inches, keeping the mudras in the hands, to make the Moshiach mudra.

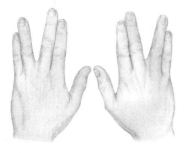 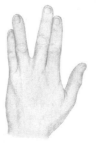 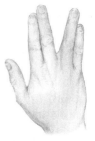

Asiyah (Tan Tien)

❖ Concentrate on the point 2 to 3
   inches below the navel and
   2 to 3 inches into the body (Tan
   Tien). Place the Shekhinah/
   Kundalini mudra.

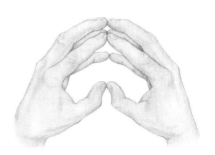

❖ Finish by looking at the Tree of Life mudras (Figure 17.1), or
place the approriate Sefirah mudra, or hold the active Sefirah point
until muscle strength return.

Appendix III

Pronunciation Guide

Hebrew letters and words can be pronounced in various ways. Ashkenazi Hebrew comes from European Jewry, whereas Sephardic Hebrew has Middle Eastern roots. Either pronunciation seems to activate the Kabbalistic patterns in this book.

Alef	a' lef	a as in father, e as in let
Beyt	bet	e as in get
Gimel	gi' mel	i as in sit, e as in met
Daleth	da' let(th)	a as in father, e as in let
Heh	heh	e as in met
Vav	vav	a as in father
Zayin	za' yin	a as in father
Chet	khet	kh is a rough throat sound, e as in get
Tet	tet	e as in get
Yod	yood	oo as in good
Caph	kaf	a as in father
Lamed	la' med	a as in father, e as in met
Mem	mem	e as in met
Nun	noon	oo as in soon
Samek	sa' mek	a as in father, e as in met
Ayin	a' yin	a as in father, yin as in bin
Pey	peh	e as in met
Tzadik	tza' deek	a as father, ee as in he
Qoof	koof	oo as in hoof

Resh	resh	e as in met
Shin	shin	i as in sin
Tau	taw	a as in father
Kether	keh' ter	e as in get, e as in get
Hokhmah	khock' mah	kh is a rough sound, o as in load, a as in father
Binah	bee nah'	ee as in bee, a as in father
Hesed	khe' sed	kh is a rough sound, both e's as in get
Gevurah	ge voo rah'	e as in met, oo as in soon, a as in father
Tifereth	tif' er et(th)	i as in bit, both e's as in get
Netzach	net' zakh	e as in get, a as in father, kh is a rough sound
Hod	hod	o as in load
Yesod	yeh sod'	e as in get, o as in load
Malkuth	mal koot(th)	a as in father, oo at in soon
B'reshith	buh ray sheeth	a as in day, e as in she
Yisrael	yis' rah ale	i as in his
Ehyeh	eh yeh'	e as in get
Ahsher	ah share'	
Shekhinah	sheh kee nah'	e as in get
Echad	eh khad'	e as in get, a as in father
Moshiach	moh shee' akh	o as in moss, a as in father
Reshith	ray sheeth'	a as in day
Tov	tove	o as in stove

Ra'a	rah' ah'	a as in father
Acharit	ah kha rit'	a as in father, i as in bit
Atziluth	at' zee looth	a as in bat
B'riyah	buh ree' yah	
Yetzirah	yet' zee rah	e as in get
Asiyah	ah see' ah	a as in father
Ajna	ajz nah	a as in father
Visuddha	vih soo dah	i as in his, a as in father
Anahata	ah nah ha tah	a as in father
Manipura	mah nee poo rah	
Svadisthana	svah deest ha nah	
Muladhara	moo lah dah rah	

Bibliography and Resources

Achad, Frater (1992). *The Anatomy of the Body of God.* Kila, MT: Kessinger Publishing.

Anonymous (1985). *Meditations on the Tarot.* Amity, NY: Amity House.

Anthony, Carol K. (1980). *A Guide to the I Ching.* Stow, MA: Anthony Publishing.

Ashlag, Yehuda (1973). *Kabbalah Ten Luminous Emanations.* New York: Research Centre of Kabbalah.

Bailey, Alice (1973). *A Treatise on Cosmic Fire.* London: Lucis Publishing.

Behmen, Jacob (1909). *The Three Principles of Divine Essence.* Chicago: Yogi Publication Society.

Belk, Henry (1974). *A Cosmic Road Map and Guide Analysis.* Self-published.

Chambers, Shirley (2000). *Kabalistic Healing.* Lincolnwood, IL: Keats Publishing.

Chia, Mantak (1984). *Taoist Secrets of Love, Cultivating Male Sexual Energy.* New York: Aurora Press.

Childre, Doc, & Martin, Howard (1999). *The Heartmath Solution.* San Francisco: HarperCollins.

De Purucker, G. (1941). *Man in Evolution,* Pasadena, CA: Theosophical Press.

Deadman, Peter, & Al-Khafiji, Mazin (1998). *A Manual of Acupuncture.* Vista, CA: Eastland Press.

Dossey, Larry, (1997). *Healing Words: The Power of Prayer and the Practice of Medicine*, New York: Harper.

Dossey, Larry (1997). *Prayer Is Good Medicine: How to Reap the Healing Benefits of Prayer.* New York: HarperCollins.

Drucker, Johanna (1995). *The Alphabetic Labyrinth.* London: Thames and Hudson Ltd.

Feldman, Daniel Hale (1984). *Clear Magic.* Petaluma, CA: Garden of YH-Light.

Feldman, Daniel Hale (2001). *Qabalah, The Mystical Heritage of the Children of Abraham* Santa Cruz, CA: Work of the Chariot.

Fuller, J.F.C. *The Secret Wisdom of the Qabalah.* London: Rider & Co.

Geuerstein, Georg (1998). *Tantra, The Path of Ecstasy.* Boston, MA: Shambhala Publications.

Glazerson, Matityahu (1991). *Letters of Fire, Mystical Insights Into the Hebrew Language.* Spring Valley, NY: Feldheim.

Godwin, Joscely (1979). *Athanasius Kircher.* New York: Thames & Hudson.

Gray, William (1977). *The Talking Tree.* York Beach, ME: Samuel Weiser.

Gray, William (1984). *Concepts of Qabalah.* York Beach, ME: Samuel Weiser.

Halevi, Z'ev ben Shimon (1974). *Adam and the Kabbalistic Tree.* York Beach, ME: Samuel Weiser.

Halevi, Z'ev ben Shimon (1978). *The Anatomy of Fate.* York Beach, ME: Samuel Weiser.

Halevi, Z'ev ben Shimon (1979). *Kabbalah, Tradition of Hidden Knowledge.* New York: Thames & Hudson.

Hall, Manly P. (1977). *An Encyclopedic Outline of Masonic, Hermetic, Qabbalistic and Rosicrucian Symbolical Philosophy.* Los Angeles: The Philosophical Research Society.

Hellinger, Bert, Weber, Gunthard, & Beaumont, Hunter (1998). *Love's Hidden Symmetry.* Phoenix, AZ: Zieg, Tucker & Co.

Hellinger, Bert (2001). *Loves Own Truths.* Phoenix, AZ: Zieg, Tucker & Co.

Hellinger, Bert (2002). *Insights.* Heidelberg, Germany: Carl-Auer-Systeme Publishers.

Hellinger, Bert, www.hellinger.com and www.hellingerusa.com.

Hewes, Gordon, W. *A History of the Study of Language Origins and the Gestural Primacy Hypothesis.* Handbook of Human Symbolic Evolution, Lock & Peters, Eds.

Hook, Diana (1973). *The I Ching and You.* New York: Dutton.

Hook, Diana (1975). *The I Ching and Mankind.* London: Routledge & Kegan Paul.

Hurtak, J.J. (1977). *The Book of Knowledge, The Keys of Enoch.* Los Gatos, CA: The Academy for Future Science.

International College of Applied Kinesiology (ICAK), www.icakusa.com.

Iverson, Jana, & Goldin-Meadow, Susan (1998). *Why People Gesture When They Speak, Nature.*

Johari, Harish (2000). *Chakras, Energy Centers of Transformation.* Rochester, VT: Destiny Books.

Kaplan, Aryeh (1974). *The Aryeh Kaplan Anthology, Vols. I & II.* Brooklyn, NY: Mesorah Publications.

Kaplan, Aryeh (1978). *Meditation and the Bible*. York Beach, ME: Samuel Weiser.

Kaplan, Aryeh (1979). *The Bahir*. York Beach, ME: Samuel Weiser.

Kaplan, Aryeh (1984). *The Chasidic Masters*. Brooklyn, NY: Moznaim Publishing.

Kaplan, Aryeh (1986). *A Call to the Infinite*. Brooklyn, NY: Moznaim Publishing.

Kaplan, Aryeh (1990). *Inner Space*. Brooklyn, NY: Moznaim Publishing

Kaplan, Aryeh (1990). *Sefer Yetzirah, The Book of Creation*. York Beach, ME: Samuel Weiser.

Kaplan, Aryeh (1993). *Immortality, Resurrection, and the Age of The Universe: A Kabbalistic View*. Hoboken, NJ: KTAV Publishing House.

Kennedy, Jan (1982). Psychoenergetics, *A Breath of Life*. San Diego, CA: Cosmoenergetics Publications.

Kenton, Rebecca, www.kabbalahsociety.org.

Khanna, Madhu (1979). *Yantra, The Tantric Symbol of Cosmic Unity*. London: Thames & Hudson.

Knight, Gareth (1978). *A Practical Guide to Qabalistic Symbolism*. York Beach, ME: Samuel Weiser.

Krakowski, Steve, http://ddi.digital.net/~krakowss/index.html.

Kushner, Lawrence (1977). *Honey From the Rock*. Woodstock, VT: Jewish Lights Publishing.

Kushner, Lawrence (2001). *The Way Into Jewish Mystical Tradition*. Woodstock, VT: Jewish Lights Publishing.

Lawlor, Robert (1982). *Sacred Geometry.* London: Thames & Hudson.

Leadbeater, C.W. (1927). *The Chakras.* Wheaton, IL: The Theosophical Publishing House.

Leet, Lenora (1999). *The Secret Doctrine of the Kabbalah.* Rochester, VT: Inner Traditions.

Levi, Eliphas (1973). *The Book of Splendor.* York Beach, ME: Samuel Weiser.

MacDonald, Michael-Albion (1986). *The Secret of Secrets.* Gillette, NJ: Heptangle Books.

Madaule, Paul (1994). *When Listening Comes Alive.* Norval, Ont.: Moulin Publishing.

Mathers, S.L. MacGregor (1968). *The Kabbalah Unveiled.* York Beach, ME: Samuel Weiser.

Maturana & Varela (1987). *The Tree of Knowledge.* Boston: Shambhala Publications.

Melchizedek, Drunvalo (1998). *The Ancient Secret of the Flower of Life.* Flagstaff, AZ: Light Technology Publishing.

Metabolics, www.metabolics.co.uk.

Mookerjee, Ajit (1982). *Kundalini, The Arousal of the Inner Energy.* Rochester, Vt.: Destiny Books.

Motoyama, Hiroshi (1981). *Theories of the Chakras.* Wheaton, IL: The Theosophical Publishing House.

Munk, Michael L. (1983). *The Wisdom of the Hebrew Alphabet.* Brooklyn, NY: Mesorah Publications.

Newberg, Andrew, D'Aquili, Eugene, & Rause, Vince (2002). *Why God Won't Go Away.* New York: Ballantine Books.

Ni, Hua Ching (1983). *The Book of Changes and Unchanging Truth.* Malibu, CA: Shrine of the Eternal Breath of Tao.

Oschman, James L. (2000). *Energy Medicine.* New York: Churchill Livingstone.

Oschman, James (1997). *What is Healing Energy? Part 2, Journal of Bodywork and Movement Therapies, 1(2),* 117-128.

Ouaknin, Marc-Alain, *Mysteries of the Kabbalah.* New York: Abbeville Press.

Paraliminal Tapes, Learning Strategies Corp., www.learningstrategies. com.

Penfield, W., & T. Rasmussen (1950). *The Cerebral Cortex of Man.* New York: Macmillan.

Pick, Bernhard (1974). *The Cabala.* La Salle, IL: Open Court.

Place, Ullin T. (2000). The Role of the Hand in the Evolution of Language. *Psycoloquy*: 11(007) Language Gesture (1).

Plummer, L. Gordon, (1982). *By the Holy Tetraktys!*, Buena Park, CA: Point Loma Publications.

Poizner, H., Klima, E., & Bellugi, U. (1987). *What the Hands Reveal about the Brain.* Cambridge, MA: MIT Press.

Ponce, Charles (1973). *Kabbalah.* Wheaton, IL: The Theosophical Publishing House.

Powell, A. E. (1969). *The Etheric Double.* Wheaton, IL: The Theosophical Publishing House.

Purce, Jill (1974). *The Mystic Spiral, Journey of the Soul.* New York: Thames & Hudson.

Raphael (1993). *Pathway of Fire.* York Beach, ME: Samuel Weiser.

Rosner, Fred (translator and editor) (1978). *Biblical and Talmudic Medicine.* Norvale, NJ: Jason Aronson.

Sannella, Lee (1976). *Kundalini, Psychosis or Transcendence?* San Francisco: H. S. Dakin.

Savedow, Steve (2000). *The Book of the Angel Rezial.* York Beach, ME: Samuel Weiser.

Schmitt, Jr., Walter, www.theuplink.com/.

Scholem, Gershom (1991). *On the Mystical Shape of the Godhead.* New York: Schocken Books.

Schonberger, Martin (1979). *The I Ching and the Genetic Code.* New York: ASI Publishers.

Schutz, Albert L. (1980). *Call Adonoi.* Goleta, CA: Quantal Publishing.

Sheldrake, Rupert (2001). Morphic Resonance and Family Constellations, *Systemic Solutions Bulletin.* London, England.

Shima, Miki (1992). *The Medical I Ching.* Boulder, CO: Blue Poppy Press.

Skinner, Ralston (1982. *The Source of Measures.* San Diego, CA: Wizards Bookshelf.

Sperling, Simon, & Levertoff translators (1984). *The Zohar.* London: Soncino Press.

Spock, Marjorie (1980). *Eurythmy.* Spring Valley, NY: The Anthroposophic Press.

Steiner, Rudolf (1982). *Genesis.* London: Rudolf Steiner Press.

Stirling, William (1981). *The Cannon*. London: Research Into Lost Knowledge Organization.

Suares, Carlo (1968). *The Sepher Yetsira*. Boston: Shambhala Publications.

Suares, Carlo (1985). *The Qabala Trilogy*. Boston: Shambhala Publications.

Sung, Z. D. (1971). *The Symbols of Yi King*. Taipei: Ch'eng Wen Publishing.

Thie, John F. (1979). Touch for Health. Los Angeles, CA: DeVorss & Company.

Tiqunim HaZohar, 1558.

Touch For Health, www.touchforhealth.com.

Walter, Katya (1994). *Tao of Chaos*. Austin, TX: Kairos Center.

Walther, David (2000). *Applied Kinesiology, 2nd Edition*. Pueblo, CO: systemsdc.

Weiner, Herbert (1969). $9^1/2$ *Mystics, The Kabbala Today*. New York: Collier Books.

Wilhelm, Baynes (1977). *The I Ching or Book of Changes*. Princeton, NJ: Princeton University Press.

Wilson, Frank R. (1998). *The Hand*. New York: Pantheon Books.

Wing, R.L. (1982). *The Illustrated I Ching*. New York: Doubleday.

Work of the Chariot, www.workofthechariot.com.

Yan, Johnson F. (1991). *DNA and the I Ching*. Berkeley, CA: North Atlantic Books.

Yogananda, Paramahansa (1946). *Autobiography of a Yogi*, Los Angeles: Self Realization Fellowship.

Yudelove, Eric Stephen (1995). *The Tao & the Tree of Life*. St. Paul, MN: Llewellyn Publications.

Index

Dale Schusterman, DC, DIBAK

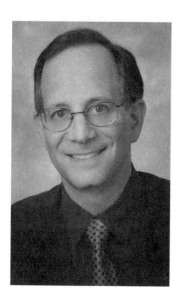

Dr. Schusterman practiced in Northern Virginia for 29 years after graduating from Logan College of Chiropractic in 1977. He is a graduate of the University of Michigan (1973) and he is a diplomate in Applied Kinesiology, which is a unique system for assessing the status of the nervous system in relation to health and the treatment of dis-ease. Dr. Schusterman also facilitates Family Constellation workshops and seminars in Sign Language of the Soul. He now lives in Chapel Hill, NC with his wife and daughter.